The Prostate Cure

THE
PROSTATE
CURE

The Revolutionary, Natural Approach

to Treating Enlarged Prostates

HARRY G. PREUSS, M.D.
BRENDA D. ADDERLY, M.H.A.

Crown Publishers, Inc.

New York

Published by Crown Publishers, Inc., 201 East 50th Street, New York, New York 10022. Member of the Crown Publishing Group.

Random House, Inc. New York, Toronto, London, Sydney, Auckland
www.randomhouse.com

CROWN is a trademark of Crown Publishers, Inc.

Printed in the United States of America

Design by Lenny Henderson

Library of Congress Cataloging-in-Publication Data
Preuss, Harry G.
     The prostate cure / Harry G. Preuss and Brenda D. Adderly.
     p. cm.
     Includes bibliographical references and index.
     (hardcover)
     1. Benign prostatic hyperplasia. 2. Flower pollen—Therapeutic use.
I. Adderly, Brenda. II. Title.
RC899.P65   1998
616.6'506—dc21   98-29437
                                                  CIP

ISBN 0-609-60323-X

10 9 8 7 6 5 4 3 2 1

First Edition

An Important Note to Our Readers

The material in this book is for informational purposes only. It is not intended to serve as a prescription for you, or to replace the advice of your medical doctor. Please discuss all aspects of the Prostate Cure with your physician *before* beginning any program. If you have any medical conditions, or are taking prescription or nonprescription medications, see your physician before altering or discontinuing the use of them.

Why do we use the word "cure"?

Our use of the word *cure* is substantiated by several references. We use the word *cure* to mean the partial or complete relief of the symptoms of an enlarged prostate. Obviously, nothing in the title or content of this book is intended to suggest that the use of the recommended supplement or program will fully reduce benign prostatic hyperplasia (BPH).

The evidence, carefully collected in this book, fully substantiates that the supplement recommended is frequently effective for long periods of time. However, we offer no guarantee that *every* individual will benefit from this program.

DEDICATION

To my family.
—HARRY PREUSS

To my husband,
Peter Engel, for his tremendous love and support
during the gestation of this book,
and to our twin sons, gestating too.
—BRENDA ADDERLY

ACKNOWLEDGEMENTS

We first owe a huge debt of gratitude to Howard Cohl, Peter Engel, Jeffry Still, Sandra Thomson, and everyone at Affinity for their support, hard work, understanding, and encouragement during this project.

Also, we would like to thank our amazing editor, Kristin Kiser, for her guidance and fortitude. She inspired us when we needed it, was patient when problems loomed, and *always* kept the faith. We are deeply grateful.

CONTENTS

Authors' Note   xiii

Chapter 1   Benign Prostatic Hyperplasia:
                    Men's Secret Disease   1

Chapter 2   Standard Non-oral Approaches
                    to Treating BPH   31

Chapter 3   Alternatives to Surgery   57

Chapter 4   The Miracle of Cernitin   79

Chapter 5   The Prostate Cure:
                    A Seven-Step Proactive Program   107

Chapter 6   Living Well Is the Best Revenge   135

Chapter 7   Prostate Cancer   165

Chapter 8   Conclusion   195

Notes   199

Appendix   229

Glossary   231

Index   245

AUTHORS' NOTE

How to Evaluate the Information in This Book

Throughout *The Prostate Cure,* we will present information from a number of studies on well-known procedures used to treat BPH (benign prostatic hyperplasia, or enlargement of the prostate) and on the studies that have accumulated using Cernitin. We think the data speaks for itself, but to help you evaluate that information on your own, we want to leave the topic of BPH for a moment and explain some of the rudiments of medical research and what is involved in various types of studies.

When a new medical product is developed, it may first be tested in the laboratory on animals, animal tissue, or human tissue (often removed during surgery) to determine its effectiveness. As you will see in Chapter 4, *laboratory research* was done many times on rats for Cernitin to determine the actual contents of the products and what components of Cernitin were doing what.

If a product appears promising and not toxic to the animals, research may progress to use with humans. Sometimes the reverse happens; that is, something that appears to be successful with humans may then be tested in the laboratory to determine why and how it works and what its chemical components are.

Anecdotal reports are often the first information the medical community has about a new product. A doctor discovers serendipitously that a product that is being used for one thing also has other results; or he discovers in some other personal way that a certain product works, as did Dr. Erik Ask-Upmark when he found that Cernitin worked for him personally. The doctor reports his personal or informal use of the product with a certain number of patients to the medical community, usually through a commentary or letter in a medical journal, and other doctors begin to look for the same results. More and more anecdotal experiences begin to accumulate, as they did with Cernitin. Typically these say something like, "We gave this product to x number of men in our practice over a period of x months, and this is what we have discovered; that is, our results agree or do not agree with those of others, and these are the side effects or difficulties (if any) we have noted."

As anecdotal reports accumulate, they pique the interest of medical researchers, who then have enough information to design a *scientific study.* Good scientific research has very specific rules, especially with regard to length of time, number of people studied, and so forth. Large sample sizes of people studies, for instance, tend to balance out the inherent differences in people, while long-term studies (conducted over several years) work to balance out natural changes that may occur over time. If these rules cannot be followed, a study may be referred to as a *pilot study,* meaning that while it suggests certain results, it was too short or did not use enough people to employ appropriate statistics. Percentages of success or change are often used in pilot studies to report results. Both pilot studies and appropriately designed scientific studies were conducted on Cernitin.

Among the other important rules for research is that of comparing the effects of a certain product against the effects of a placebo (a sham product known to have no effect). The placebo has to be of the same size, shape, etc., as the product, so that neither the person giving it nor the person taking it knows whether he or she is getting the placebo or the tested product. This is called a *double-blind* study (both people are "blind" as to who is receiving what) and reduces the introduction of bias into the investigation. The first double-blind study using Cernitin was conducted in 1962.

Sometimes the researchers know who is receiving the tested product and who is receiving the placebo. This is a *single-blind* study, considered not quite as scientific since those who know might conceivably have a vested interest in the results coming out a certain way. Randomizing the groups helps to avoid this.

Randomization means that when someone agrees to participate in the study, they have an equal chance of being selected for either group. That chance can be as simple as tossing a coin (heads for treatment; tails for placebo), although there are other more sophisticated and complicated ways to determine randomization.

You can readily see that if each person has an equal chance of belonging to either group, then randomized groups typically have close to the same number of persons. The two groups do not usually turn out to be exactly the same, however. Beware the randomized study that says there were 23 people in the treatment group and 23 in the placebo group. Typically this does not happen, although if one group starts with 25, say, and another with 23, and two people drop out of the first group, it is possible to end up with an equal number of participants in each group.

Various physical tests (e.g., blood, urine), questionnaires, and/or attitudinal measures are taken before and after the research period (and sometimes during), and the results are compared via statistics. Sometimes you will read in our report of a study that certain before/after or between group numbers (data) "differed significantly" or that the differences "were statistically significant" (we have used both terms interchangeably). This means that the researchers used certain statistical computations to show that the *differences* or the *changes* could not have occurred by chance and the supposition is, therefore, that they occurred as a result of the product being tested. While a certain range of numbers may look like an important change at first glance, if they are not statistically significant, they fall within the realm of changes that could have simply occurred by chance, not as a result of the procedure or product being tested.

As you read the research in this book you will come across words like "Boyarsky," "symptom indices," and "IPSS." These refer to systems for categorizing symptoms and their severity, and changes in these symptoms or "scores" indicate a worsening or lessening of BPH symptoms. One of the first attempts to provide guidelines for the evaluation and treatment of BPH was created in 1977 by Dr. S. Boyarsky and his colleagues; results of these evaluations are often referred to in research studies as "Boyarsky scores."[1] In 1983 a second set of guidelines was developed as part of a system for selecting candidates for prostate surgery. It was known as the Madsen-Iversen Symptom Severity Index.

Because there were problems in understanding the wording and administration of both the Boyarsky and Madsen-Iversen devices, the American Urological Association (AUA) developed a symptom index, which is used extensively to determine the success of both research and treatment.[2] Its primary function is to provide an outcome measurement to be used in evaluating the alternative treatment options, and it is one of the most widely used measurements of BPH severity.

The BPH symptom index developed by the AUA assigns a score to individuals based on the severity (from 0 to 5) of seven key symptoms: urgency, daytime and nighttime urinary frequency, hesitancy, intermittency, sensation of incomplete emptying of the bladder, and force of urine stream. A man with a total score of 0 to 7 is said to have mild symptoms. A score of 8 to 19 indicates moderate symptoms, while a score of 20 to 35 indicates severe symptoms (see the Appendix for a copy of the AUA symptom index).[3]

In 1991, after the International Consensus on Urological Diseases recommended that BPH be compared in different regions using the same case definition, the AUA symptom index was adopted by the group and renamed the International Prostate Symptom Score (IPSS).[4]

Another prominent test used to assess the effectiveness of treatment and research programs is *urinary flow rate,* often presented as the *peak* or *maximum flow rate.* A number of quality-of-life questionnaires are being, or have been, developed in order to add this measure to BPH research, and you will read about it as a category in some of our research reports. To help in the future comparison of epidemiological and clinical trials with BPH throughout the world, a nine-item Quality of Life scale was recently developed in France and is currently undergoing translation and testing in the United Kingdom, Italy, The Netherlands, Germany, Spain, Portugal, Denmark, Sweden, Norway, and the United States.[5]

Finally, when enough information (laboratory analyses, symptom indices, quality of life information) from good research has been acquired to determine that a new product or procedure looks viable, a large group of doctors at a number of clinics across the United States will participate in *clinical trials,* giving the drug or using the procedure until additional information has been acquired over a long enough period of time to show the short- and long-term effects of the drug/procedure on a variety of persons. Only after clinical trials are completed, can the pharmaceutical manufacturer of a new drug apply for approval of the drug by the Federal Drug Administration (FDA).

1

BENIGN PROSTATIC HYPERPLASIA (BPH): MEN'S SECRET DISEASE

What, exactly, is the prostate and what does it do?

*

What is benign prostatic hyperplasia or BPH?

*

What are the symptoms of BPH?

*

What causes BPH?

*

What role do hormones play in BPH?

*

When does a man begin to be affected by BPH?

*

What is the difference between BPH and cancer of the prostate?

*

Can BPH turn into prostate cancer?

It begins so gradually and imperceptibly that you may not even notice it. You visit the rest room several more times than usual during the workday—maybe you're just drinking more water. You interrupt business meetings for a "bathroom break" more often than your colleagues—it could just be the stress of your job that

makes you anxious. But you also haven't sat through an entire con-
cert or movie for years, and when you fly you always ask for an aisle
seat so as not to disturb fellow passengers with your frequent trips
to the bathroom. It's slightly annoying and more than a bit embarrassing, but not cause for major concern. Or so you think.

At night, though, you begin to realize that something has
changed. Your sleep is interrupted by bathroom calls as often as
every two or three hours. Being awakened four times per night—and
feeling lousy every day because of sleep deprivation—does make
you a bit worried and confused. Is it stress, your diet, or too many
beers after work? Looking for a medical answer, you may attribute
your difficulties to a shrinking bladder—but in fact this condition
has nothing to do with the bladder. Instead, this *increased frequency
of the need to urinate* is probably the first noticeable and major sign
of a growing prostate, called by doctors benign prostatic hyperplasia (BPH), and more commonly referred to by the public as an
"enlarged prostate" (hyperplasia means "an enlargement due to an
increased number of cells").

> *BPH is as common a part of aging as graying hair.
> One doctor calls it the "gift" of maturity.[1]*

BPH is a secret, silent disease. Silent because men commonly
don't feel its progression, and secret because men who have it—
and most will during their lifetime—don't talk about it. Nevertheless, it's so prevalent that comedians frequently joke about the
symptoms ("a good night is one in which you only have to get up
once"). The symptoms run the gamut from merely annoying, to
downright uncomfortable, to, in the worst-case scenario, totally
excruciating.

It has been estimated that the annual costs of treating men for BPH exceeds $4 billion.[2]

THE NUMBER ONE BENIGN TUMOR IN MEN

Benign prostatic hyperplasia is *the most common* noncancerous (benign means "nonmalignant") tumor in men and ranks with prostate cancer as the two most common prostate disorders affecting middle-aged and older men. (More about prostate cancer in Chapter 7.) Currently some 10 million American men exhibit signs of BPH, and of these, 5.6 million men may need treatment for it—a statistic that could double by the year 2020, as the male population ages and significantly impacts the health care system.[3] Although doctors and research scientists have several theories about how BPH develops, the truth is that they have yet to fully understand why it occurs.

What we do know (from autopsy studies of men who died from causes other than prostate enlargement) is that a man's prostate typically starts to enlarge at about age 45, although about 10 percent of men between the ages of 25 to 30 years also have BPH.[4] By age 50, about half of all men will have some noticeable signs of the disease. The number rises to 60 percent at age 60 and continues to escalate over the next two and a half decades, until by the time they reach 85 years of age, 90 percent of all men suffer significant symptoms. In other words, if they live long enough, nearly all men will develop at least microscopic evidence of BPH.[5]

Interestingly, BPH does not distinguish between race or nationality, although African-American men are at a slightly greater risk than white American males.[6] The condition also does not seem to be related to sexual activity or the lack thereof, since it occurs in celibate priests with the same frequency as sexually active men—and is also not related to either sexual excesses or deprivation.[7]

Although BPH may be inevitable for most men, the annoying symptoms don't have to be. At no other time in history have so many good treatment options been available, and never before have so many men actively sought out these options. Rest assured that reading *The Prostate Cure* is an excellent first step towards seeking—and finding—relief for the symptoms of BPH.

THE ROLE OF THE PROSTATE GLAND

One medical expert, Dr. Stephen N. Rous, notes that the prostate generates "more questions, more misunderstandings, more concern, and more anxieties than any other part of the male genitourinary tract."[8] This small gland at the base of the bladder causes more grief for men than just about any other structure of their bodies, and difficulties with it can cover almost the entire adult life of a man.[9] Yet many men rarely think about their prostates, and in fact, until trouble begins, many may not even know where it is or what it does.

When a baby boy is born, his prostate is about the size of a pea, and it thereafter grows slowly until reaching almond-size at the

An article in the March 26, 1995 edition of the London Times indicated that 89 percent of men asked did not know where their prostate gland was, while some 62 percent mistook it for the bladder. Only half of the men knew that only males have a prostate.[10]

onset of puberty. Under the influence of sex hormones, the prostate then begins a stage of more rapid, continual growth until a man reaches his late 20s or early 30s, by which time it is about the size of a walnut or large chestnut and weighs a little less than an ounce.[11]

Partly glandular and partly composed of smooth muscle tissue, the prostate surrounds the neck of the bladder and wraps around the urethra (the thin channel leading from the bladder through the penis, and through which both urine and sperm pass from the body). Because the prostate is only indirectly involved in procreation, it is considered an accessory rather than a key part of the male repro-ductive system, but it nevertheless is a particularly vulnerable part of the male anatomy.

To help visualize this, think of the prostate as a fist holding a straw (the urethra). Beginning somewhere around age 40, cells in most men's prostate commence to multiply again, and they continue to do so slowly until death. The enlarged tissue of the prostate is like the fist squeezing the straw, thereby making it difficult for urine to pass through the urethra. In severe cases the prostate can grow to up to 10 times its normal size.[12] (In a relatively few men, however, the prostate actually shrinks or atrophies during their later years.)

As late as the 1970s, researchers were still unsure of the prostate's role in the body. Although many small glands within the prostate secrete several different substances, we know now that its key function is to produce and discharge the viscid, alkaline fluid that comprises a major portion of the seminal fluid. The prostatic fluid helps to maintain an appropriate environment in which sperm can live; provides them with some nourishment; and, in general, increases their survival time after ejaculation.

The prostatic fluid also contains prostaglandins—hormone-like fatty acids that affect smooth muscle fibers and blood vessel walls. One of the many theories about the prostaglandins produced by the prostate is that they encourage the cervix (the entrance to the female uterus) to dilate, thus enabling sperm to pass through it and fertilize the egg.[13]

Tiny chambers within the glandular tissue of the prostate make and store prostatic fluid more or less continuously. During ejaculation, the muscles in the prostate contract, pushing the fluid through special ducts into the urethra; however the prostate is never totally emptied. Sperm, produced in the testes, also enter the urethra, via a tube called the vas deferens. With ejaculation, the sperm, prostatic fluid, and other fluids combine to carry the sperm out of the body.

Although there are no actual, observable demarcations within the prostate itself, doctors often speak of it as being made up of five "lobes" or "zones": an anterior lobe, posterior lobe, two lateral lobes, and a middle lobe. The anterior consists mainly of smooth muscle and occupies about 30 percent of the tiny gland.

The part of the prostate that surrounds the urethra is considered the middle lobe and is sometimes called the central zone. It is enveloped by larger, peripheral zones on either side of the urethra. These zones are composed primarily (about 75 percent) of glands, which are usually the primary sites where cancer develops, although cancer of the periurethral ducts can arise in the central zone.

A small transitional zone lies within the middle lobe, adjacent to the urethral sphincter, and *is the sole site of benign prostatic hyperplasia.*[14] Before enlargement, this small transition zone comprises only 2 percent of the entire mass of a normal prostate gland.[15]

As the tissue in the transitional zone grows, true prostate tissue is displaced and the prostate gland gradually becomes grossly enlarged. The new growth is composed of the same general type of tissue as the normal prostate, except that it is more fibrous and muscular in nature.[16] The growth typically occurs in an asymmetrical manner, extending most of the way or part of the way around the prostatic urethra (that part of the urethra surrounded by the prostate), and begins to constrict the urethra. The effects of BPH on

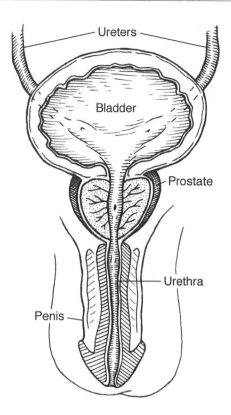

Figure 1.1 Cross section of the prostate, bladder, and urethra
The prostate, a muscular, walnut-shaped gland, is actually only about an inch and a half long, yet it can cause much trouble.

the urethra can vary, depending on the nature of the growth. If it enlarges in a primarily outward direction, for example, the prostate can reach a huge size, relatively speaking, yet not cause any significant obstructive symptoms of the urethra. Accordingly, some men with greatly enlarged prostates experience little or no obstruction; whereas some relatively small prostates produce severe obstruction.[17]

The prostate plays no direct role in the functioning of the male's urinary system, but because it is situated so close to the bladder and the urethra, when it goes awry, a myriad of urinary problems can

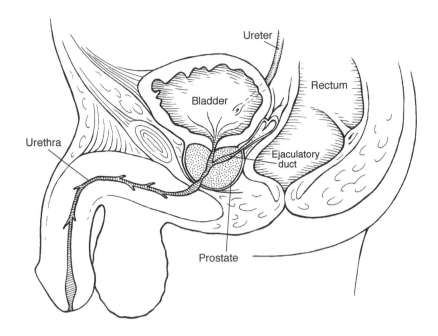

Figure 1.2 Side view of the prostate

The prostate completely encircles the urethra, so as a man ages and his prostate grows, the urethra becomes constricted, making it difficult for urine to pass out of the body.

result. In fact, BPH symptoms occur primarily because enlargement of the prostate constricts the urethra and obstructs urinary flow. Prostatic infection also can result in painful or burning urination.

THE SYMPTOMS OF BPH

Referring to his need to urinate several times each night, one man with BPH told us that "I haven't had a full night's sleep in 10 years, nor a morning that isn't gray with fatigue." The number of times that men are awakened during the night varies with the degree of urinary obstruction; however, in severe cases, it may occur hourly.[18]

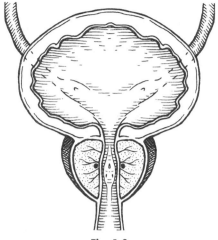

Fig. 1.3

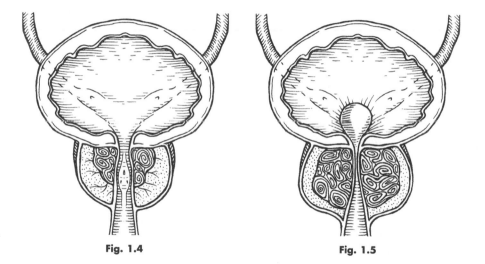

Fig. 1.4   Fig. 1.5

Figure 1.3 to 1.5 The many shapes of BPH

In Figure 1.3 you can see that BPH (the small black dot) begins in the smallest—yet most strategically placed—area of the prostate, the transition zone. In Figure 1.4, which illustrates an early phase of BPH, nodules have begun to form, as cell growth causes prostate enlargement. In Figure 1.5, the lateral lobes have enlarged and constricted the urethra, a condition that often results in the obstruction of urine flow.

> *The fatigue that results from frequent awakening during the night is only one of the side effects of the obstructive symptoms of BPH.*

The disconcerting feeling of needing to urinate *even after having done so* is a second major symptom of BPH. Only minutes after urinating, a man may experience the sensation that his bladder is not empty and that he needs to urinate again. This occurs because the enlarging prostate pushes on the bottom of the bladder and reduces its capacity to hold urine; hence, the increased frequency, and the signaling of a false need for urination. Another, related, cause is that residual urine from a not-completely-emptied bladder reduces the bladder's functional capacity. Think of a gallon jug that is never less than half-full: The jug must be emptied every half-gallon—twice as often.

Many men with BPH experience *difficulty in urinating*. This symptom is so common that author Michael Korda describes it as one of the "better-known humiliations of the aging process in men."[19] Men who are busy, traveling, or otherwise occupied may not have the opportunity to urinate the moment they feel the need, especially if the need occurs with great frequency. If they "hold it" for more than a few minutes after that first urge, however, they may experience an involuntary burst of urine. More commonly, their entire urinary system may seem to "close down," and they may barely be able to start the urinary stream. (Doctors term this delay "hesitancy.") When this happens, they may spend what seem like endless minutes standing at the toilet, pushing and straining to force the urine out, and sometimes having to repeat the process several times until a normal flow is regained. During this time they may have a urinary stream that barely dribbles despite the sense that the bladder is full. Why hesitancy occurs is not clear, but it may be due to the time it takes to attain sufficient pressure within the bladder to overcome the resistance caused by the obstructing prostate.[20]

In extreme cases of difficulty with urination—what the medical world calls "acute complete urinary retention"—a man may have to go to a hospital for emergency catheterization. This is rare and is unlikely to occur unexpectedly, but when it does happen it is clearly a physically painful and emotionally disturbing situation, not to mention inconvenient.

Another common symptom of BPH is *dribbling at the end of urination.* Doctors call this "intermittency," but men know it more intimately as that embarrassing dark spot on their trousers that appears uncontrollably after they have zipped up. It occurs because as the prostatic obstruction grows, the bladder can't empty completely with a single muscle contraction. Seconds later, however, the muscle involuntarily contracts a second time, and a small stream of urine—ranging from a few drops to an ounce or more—escapes.

Taken together, these common symptoms of BPH are called *prostatism.* Although BPH is their most frequent cause, other disorders, such as prostate or bladder infections, can also produce the same collection of symptoms. At their worst, these symptoms may signal

---

*Episodes of "acute complete urinary retention"—
extreme difficulty with urination—can result when
a person can't get to the bathroom; from
exposure to cold; from using certain anesthetic
agents, decongestants and antihistamines;
or from drinking alcohol.*

prostate cancer. But remember: *BPH is not prostate cancer, and having it doesn't mean that a man is any more likely to get prostate cancer than someone who is not so affected.*

LONG-RANGE PHYSICAL DIFFICULTIES
RELATED TO BPH

Where BPH frequently results in incomplete urine elimination, it can lead to bladder infections and cystitis (inflammation), with unpleasant symptoms that range from burning during urination to constant severe pain. While these side effects of BPH are curable with antibiotics, they are likely to recur frequently, creating another costly, inconvenient and pain-filled experience.

Because stagnant urine is an almost ideal fluid for nurturing the growth of bacteria, incomplete bladder emptying causes a circular effect in which the bladder's inability to discharge urine (called "stasis") predisposes the upper urinary tract and bladder to infections.[21] Inflammation from these infections can lead to tissue changes, usually a thickening of the tissue, which is considered by some as the cause of many of the more bothersome symptoms of BPH.[22] Bacteria growing in the urine tend to make it highly alkaline, which can also lead to the formation of stones in the bladder with, once again, severe pain and discomfort. Since they tend to gravitate toward the neck of the bladder, the stones may sometimes cause an obstruction there. They can also pass through the neck of the bladder and become lodged in the urethra, and, if they continue to pass through, cause extreme pain with their passage.

When the bladder has to work harder and contract more forcefully to expel urine, its inner surface becomes thick and irregular, a condition known as "trabeculation." This irregular thickening leaves areas of weakness in the lining of the bladder, which may extend outward to form small pouches, called "diverticula." These pockets may not drain properly, causing stones to form within them.

At its extreme, BPH can lead to full *incontinence,* where a man no longer has control over his bladder's functioning. He may not even be able to sense when he is urinating, making the wearing of adult diapers an uncomfortable and often embarrassing necessity.

Sustained or prolonged obstruction due to BPH can result in more severe conditions such as development of kidney stones, as well as bladder and kidney damage, which in turn may result in life-threatening renal failure and an excess of urea in the blood.

THE PSYCHOLOGICAL EFFECTS OF BPH

The psychological effects of BPH can be devastating. When men sense that their sexual organs are starting to fail, they can become severely depressed. The emotions that accompany balding, graying hair, or an expanding waistline do not compare to the feelings of impending powerlessness and debility that men may experience upon finding that their genitals are no longer able to even function properly for such a basic task as urination.

As BPH progresses, urinary leakage may reach the point of embarrassment, or a man may become frustrated that he needs to strain so much every time he has to urinate. Urinary frequency may be so severe that it causes a man to change his lifestyle by staying close to home and avoiding situations that make it difficult for him to urinate every hour or so. At the worst, he may have to curtail travel or vacation plans, especially long automobile rides.

Author Michael Korda relates how, when his own intermittent prostate difficulties increased, he would have to plot his course through midtown Manhattan to "take advantage of the men's rooms in hotel lobbies or department stores." Korda learned where all the

> *Many men begin to experience sexual difficulties*
> *as an indirect result of BPH—likely because the*
> *repeated need to urinate, coupled with the constant*
> *feelings of "needing to go," plus concern about*
> *urine escape, create a situation that is hardly*
> *conducive to sexual romance.*

restrooms were in public buildings and discovered that some shops would let him use the employees' toilet if he spent enough money. He developed a "fetish" for sitting in aisle seats in the movies, so that he could go to the bathroom without having to bother others.[23] Korda also describes the shame, guilt, and fear he experienced during one agonizing late-night, wintertime drive from his home outside the city to his apartment in Manhattan, where he worked. Gas station bathrooms were closed and locked, and Korda ended up parking his car illegally every 10 to 15 minutes and climbing over frozen snow banks in his street shoes in order to urinate.

THE TRIP TO THE DOCTOR

The obvious and painful symptoms delineated in the preceding paragraphs generally become progressively more difficult to ignore. If you are experiencing some or all of them, their presence may indicate that you have BPH. But to rule out prostate cancer or other prostate problems, you should undergo testing which will confirm BPH. One common test is the digital rectal exam (DRE), which involves the doctor inserting a lubricated, gloved finger up a man's rectum to the point where the doctor can feel the prostate through the wall of the rectum. A normal prostate feels smooth and elastic, while an enlarged prostate may have a rubbery consistency. Size can be misleading, however, inasmuch as a prostate that is small by rectal examination can still be sufficiently enlarged to cause obstruction. Treatment options for BPH depend, of course, not on size but on the severity of the disease for the person involved. Doctors sometimes refer to this as the "degree of bothersomeness" that BPH produces.

One procedure sometimes used in the diagnosis of BPH, especially if there's blood in the urine, is a cystoscopy. A slender, hollow tube (called a cystoscope) with lights and a lens on one end and a viewing lens on the other is passed through the opening of the anesthetized penis and threaded through the urethra and then into the bladder. It allows the doctor to search these areas for abnormalities, to determine how much obstruction of the urethra is caused by an enlarged prostate, to estimate the size and weight of the obstructing tissue, and to assess how much urine is retained in the bladder because it can't get through.[24]

Blood in the urine, or hematuria, can develop when the urethral blood vessels and the bladder neck get so stretched by the growing prostate that they burst. BPH is one of the two most common causes of hematuria in men over 40; bladder cancer is the other.[25]

THREE OTHER PROSTATE DISORDERS WITH SIMILAR SYMPTOMS

Complicating the issue of diagnosing BPH from its symptoms is the fact that all of the symptoms described in this chapter can also be indicative of three other common problems associated with the prostate: (1) bacterial infection with accompanying inflammation, (2) nonbacterial inflammation, and (3) prostate cancer. Because the treatment for each of these three conditions is quite different, a correct diagnosis is imperative.

PROSTATITIS

The first two conditions just noted can take several often confusing forms. One of these—prostatitis (a general term that denotes inflammation of the prostate)—is considered the most common urologic disease in men, yet is still considered a "poorly defined group of syndromes."[26] It afflicts between 25 to 50 percent of all adult men. With the exception of *acute bacterial prostatitis,* in which patients have a true bacterial infection that can be treated with antibiotics, it is a complex, puzzling condition because of the undetermined cause and treatment of three additional diagnostic categories subsumed under the listing of prostatitis. The first two are *chronic bacterial prostatitis,* and *nonbacterial (or abacterial) prostatitis.* In the latter, patients have symptoms and signs of prostatitis that are localized to the prostate, but no bacteria are found in the urine or in lab tests; hence, treatment with antibiotics is ineffective and unwarranted. In about 40 percent of these cases, there is, nevertheless, an increase in white blood cells in the prostatic fluid.[27]

The remaining subcategory of prostatitis is what many urologists call *prostatodynia*—though others say this and nonbacterial prostatitis are the same (more about that controversy below).[28] Whatever it is called, some experts believe prostatodynia constitutes more than half of all cases of prostatitis.[29]

ACUTE BACTERIAL PROSTATITIS

Although prostatic infection typically begins in the prostate, it can also start in some other part of the body (most likely in the prostatic urethra, that part of the urethra within the prostate) and then spread to the prostate. Bacterial prostatitis can develop when bacteria from the colon get into the prostate, usually through anal intercourse. It is not contagious nor can it be transmitted to the man's sexual partner, but the symptoms will probably not be conducive to having sex anyway.

Acute bacterial prostatitis, which results from a sudden infusion of bacteria into the prostate, comes on quickly and tends to have all or some of the following symptoms: fever, chills, malaise, aches and pains like those of the flu, low abdominal or low back pain, difficulty in urinating due to swelling of the prostate gland, and painful ejaculations.[30] While acute bacterial prostatitis is the easiest type of prostatitis to diagnose, it is the least common form of prostatitis.[31]

Acute prostatic infections and inflammation tend to occur more frequently in younger men, and can be quite painful and troublesome, as the preceding symptoms indicate. Untreated, they can also lead to far more serious disorders. An infected prostate can swell and block the flow of urine, causing a backup in the bladder. Subsequently, the bladder can become infected and pass the infection on to the kidneys.

When a prostate has enlarged to the point where the bladder cannot empty completely, bacteria can also grow in the stagnant urine that remains. Usually this is more likely to lead to a bladder infection, which can sometimes spread to the prostate. Transmittal of gonorrhea and yeast during sexual intercourse can also lead to bacterial prostatitis.

Unfortunately, the blood-prostate barrier, by which the body defenses keep certain substances from penetrating the prostate, can also keep out antibiotics, making prostatitis extremely difficult to cure. The good news is that the barrier frequently breaks down during bacterial prostatitis, allowing the antibiotics to enter after all.[32] Because of the difficulty in eradicating acute bacterial prostatitis, a

minimum of 30 days of treatment with antibiotics is frequently recommended.[33]

CHRONIC BACTERIAL PROSTATITIS

Chronic bacterial prostatitis is the name given to recurring infections of the prostate, which are likely the result of the residual infection that remains when acute bacterial prostatitis hasn't been
completely cured.[34] It may or may not produce the symptoms of
acute bacterial prostatitis, but appears usually in less dramatic and
more subtle ways.[35]

Less severe than its acute version, chronic bacterial prostatitis is,
nevertheless, the cause of recurring urinary infections and ongoing
pain for many men. Symptoms include pain that radiates into the
groin, testes, or penis; painful ejaculation; intermittent bladder irritative symptoms, such as a frequent and urgent need to urinate; and,
sometimes, a burning sensation upon urination.[36] Treatment is ineffective for a high percentage of patients with chronic prostatitis,
both from bacterial and nonbacterial causes. Sometimes called
"prostatostasis," nonbacterial inflammation is the most common
type of prostatitis and is thought by some doctors to be caused by
engorgement of the prostate's fluid-producing glands due to irregular or infrequent ejaculation.

THE CONFUSION BETWEEN PROSTATODYNIA, STRESS PROSTATITIS, AND NONBACTERIAL PROSTATITIS

In 1988 Henry C. Miller, M.D., then chairman of the Department of
Urology at George Washington University, Washington, D.C., renamed a condition that had baffled urologists for years. His diagnosis still remains controversial. Dr. Miller called the disorder "stress

> *Studies of urological literature show that various doctors and researchers often use one or more of the three terms (prostatodynia, stress prostatitis, and nonbacterial prostatitis) as synonyms for the same disorder, leaving one doctor to refer to prostatodynia as a "wastebasket" syndrome of miscellaneous pains, aches, and pelvic discomforts.[37]*

prostatitis," and at the time of his article he had identified as many as 218 men with the condition.[38]

Dr. Miller's work was one of the first to identify the prostate as a target organ for stress. He believed that stimulation of the prostate by the autonomic nerve fibers that it contains—which are known to cause stress-related symptoms in the stomach, colon, and blood vessels—results in prostatic fluid secretion and contraction of the muscular fibers within the prostate.[39]

In the years since Dr. Miller's first report, other physicians have elected to call the condition "prostatodynia,"[40] and still others have linked it with chronic nonbacterial prostatitis, a condition often described in words similar to those used by Philadelphia researchers: "ill-understood and difficult-to-diagnose."[41]

Dr. Miller believed the symptoms of stress prostatitis, which are somewhat similar to other forms of prostatitis (especially those of nonbacterial prostatitis—hence part of the confusion), occur because of changes in the prostate brought about by stress. Other reports in the literature attribute the pain of prostatodynia—if, indeed, they are the same—to muscle spasms in the neck of the bladder, the prostatic urethra, the perineum, or the pelvic floor,[42] from an inflammation in one or more of the pelvic bones, or from a disease process in the rectum.[43] Whatever the condition's source, it is clear that upon examination individuals with the condition typically have no demonstrable abnormalities of the prostate gland.[44]

By whatever name it's called, a major symptom of the condition is discomfort, with aching or pain in the genitalia, lower abdomen just above the pubic hair line, pelvis, perineum (the area between the scrotum and the anus), or prostate, generally at the end of urination. Other symptoms may include low back pain, discomfort on ejaculation, and urinary frequency. A thin, watery, early-morning urethral discharge, accompanied, naturally, by feelings of anxiety, worry, guilt, and anger, is another symptom.[45]

Too often laboratory tests and diagnostic procedures produce negative results. This is another reason the condition is often linked with nonbacterial prostatitis, for which a specific causative agent usually cannot be identified, meaning that therapy for men with the disorder is usually unsatisfactory.[46]

Dr. Miller's treatment includes reassurance, an explanation of the conditions, and stress management techniques. In a personal communication to Dr. Hernando Salcedo, Dr. Miller reported that of the 400 patients he has seen with this diagnosis, 89 percent have shown significant improvement.[47]

Since Dr. Miller's first report, other urologists have begun developing new treatment procedures, in general not distinguishing too clearly between nonbacterial prostatitis and prostatodynia. For instance, in the early 1990s, a group of doctors in Israel treated 45 men with "chronic abacterial prostatitis or prostatodynia" (identifying them as the same) with six weekly, one-hour sessions of local deep microwave hyperthermia to the prostate. All patients had failed to respond to a variety of conventional treatments administered over several years by various specialists. Twenty-five percent now experienced a complete eradication of symptoms; 50 percent had a partial response; while 25 percent showed no improvement.[48]

At the Okayama University Medical School in Japan, 36 men with nonbacterial prostatitis or prostatodynia (again, lumped into the same group) who had a long history of the condition and failure to respond to conventional treatment underwent five weekly, one-hour sessions of transrectal microwave hyperthermia to the prostate. (This procedure is detailed in Chapter 2.) Excellent results were obtained for 11 (30.6 percent) of the men, good results for 8 (22.2 percent), fair results for 8 more, and poor results for the remaining 9 (25.2 percent). Five of the men experienced minor complications (anal pain, blood in the semen and urine).[49]

Recently, a group of doctors at Kingston General Hospital in Kingston, Ontario, Canada, also used a randomized, double-blind, sham-controlled trial of transurethral microwave thermotherapy on 20 patients with nonbacterial prostatitis. Although the results are encouraging, the number of persons used in the trial were quite small, as with the preceding studies. The thermotherapy consisted of a single one-hour treatment, while sham therapy involved a session of the same length of time with the same device, but using sham software.

The researchers report that all sham-treated patients experienced some discomfort during the catheterization and treatment phase and believed that they had received actual thermotherapy. Both the patient and the evaluating urologist were "blinded" as to the actual therapy performed; that is, they did not know which patient was receiving which therapy. In phase 1 of the study, all patients were assessed three months after treatment. In phase 2, all patients from phase 1 who did not show significant improvement after initial therapy were offered a second treatment and all "sham" patients were offered an actual thermotherapy treatment. Four patients who received thermotherapy in phase 1 and all 10 patients in the sham group elected to do so. They were again evaluated after three months.

Patients were assessed using a symptom severity index and symptom frequency questionnaire, and long-term follow-up of the responder group averaged 21 months. The seven responders in the treatment group had a significant improvement in subjective global assessment of greater than 50 percent and continued to improve during the 21-month period. The treated group did better than the sham group, and 50 percent of the sham group had a favorable response after subsequent thermotherapy.[50]

According to a research summary presented in *Acta Urologica Japan,* a group of Asian doctors at the Fujigaoka Hospital, which is associated with the School of Medicine at Showa University in Japan, have been fairly successful in using low-wave frequency electrical acupuncture to treat 17 patients with chronic prostatitis. The clinical efficacy of long-term treatment was considered excellent in 30 percent and moderate in 70 percent of the patients. Following treatment, Chinese medicines and "chemical agents" were withdrawn completely for 50 percent of the patients, chemical agents were withdrawn in 30 percent, and the dose of either type of medication was reduced in the remaining 20 percent of the cases.[51]

While doctors are not rushing to apply the "stress prostatitis" to certain conditions, they are beginning to recognize that many men with chronic prostatitis who are difficult to treat with standard antibiotics also have psychological problems that contribute to the cause of the situation or to its continuation. One Seattle study found that these included relationship problems (likely related to disruptions in sexual functioning), and major depression.[52] Another study found that depression and psychosocial distress, as measured by the Minnesota Multiphasic Personality Inventory (MMPI), a well-known psychological test, were common only in 43 percent of chronic prostatitis patients who were tested.[53]

A study conducted in The Netherlands found the scores on a personality inventory and a depression inventory to be higher—

although not of great magnitude—for 50 chronic prostatitis patients than for a similar group of men who were going to have vasectomies. In this study the researchers were unable to separate out any personality variables that specifically identified chronic prostatitis patients.[54]

If, however, these kinds of studies continue to appear in the medical literature, it may well be that in the near future they will lead to more careful evaluations of chronic nonbacterial prostatitis—or whatever doctors are going to call it—and attention to the sickness-related dysfunctions accompanying it.[55] This in turn suggests that counseling and medications for depression will come to play a role in the comprehensive approach to patients with this mysterious disorder.[56]

More recently, a urologist and a clinical psychologist teamed together to conclude that chronic nonbacterial prostatitis has all the hallmarks of the chronic pain syndrome: pain as a primary complaint; a low correspondence between symptoms and medical findings; and a history of multiple, unsuccessful treatments.[57] Their research team is working to clarify the distinction between the symptoms of patients with BPH and those with chronic nonbacterial prostatitis. They have found that patients with chronic nonbacterial prostatitis reported more perineal, lower abdominal, testicular, penile, and ejaculatory pain than patients with BPH.[58]

Whether they call it nonbacterial prostatitis or prostatodynia, doctors are coming close to (but still skirting around) the issue of psychological and stress factors associated with this poorly defined, difficult-to-treat disorder.

If the chronic pain syndrome is accepted as common to chronic nonbacterial prostatitis, it means that the multitude of experience acquired from the management of other chronic pain syndromes (i.e., back pain, headaches) in using a multidisciplinary approach (including stress management) may finally prove more effective for chronic nonbacterial prostatitis than other approaches.

MISCELLANEOUS CAUSES

All or many of the symptoms described in this chapter for BPH can also be caused by urethral stricture or scarring, bladder problems, diabetes, and even neurological disorders, all of which need to be ruled out by diagnostic tests. It is estimated that about one-third of the men who are told their incontinence is due to BPH subsequently discover from lab tests (urinalysis and urine culture) and urodynamic studies (tests of urine flow and the amount of residual urine in the bladder) that an altogether different condition is the cause.[59]

PROSTATE CANCER

Prostate cancer is one of two of the most common cancers in American men (skin cancer is the other) and is the second-most-common cause of death from malignancy (lung cancer ranks first).[60] In addition to exhibiting all of the symptoms suggested in this chapter, cancer may have the added symptom of extreme fatigue and/or continuous pain in the lower back, pelvis, or upper thighs. A significant number of men with prostate cancer also have BPH, and the symptoms of BPH may in fact be what first leads them to seek medical attention.

In other situations, a man with prostate cancer may have no detectable cancer, but it will be discovered on microscopic examination of the material removed for BPH.[61] Since we will devote an entire chapter to prostate cancer (see Chapter 7), we only mention prostate cancer briefly in this chapter to point out how the symptoms of advanced cancer may mimic the symptoms of BPH.

WHY DOES BPH DEVELOP?

Like prostate cancer, no one really knows what causes BPH, although the two are not linked otherwise. Having BPH does not lead to prostate cancer, and while prostate cancer can result in an enlarged prostate, it is not BPH. If a man has a partial prostatectomy or removal of prostate tissue for BPH (see Chapter 2), any prostate tissue remaining is as capable as ever of developing cancer.

The prostate is regulated by sex hormones called androgens. The most commonly known of these is testosterone, which is manufactured in the testes but actually controlled by a hormone in the pituitary gland called the luteinizing hormone-releasing hormone (LH-RH). Testosterone that has been released from the testes circu-

> *Based on the amounts of certain enzymes and hormones found in BPH tissue, researchers speculate there may be several sets of factors that stimulate the growth of the prostate in BPH. In any case, the condition is clearly related to the presence of circulating male hormones and to aging.*

lates in the blood and enters the prostate by diffusion through cell membranes, where it is transformed by the enzyme 5-alpha-reductase into dihydrotestosterone (dy-hy-dro-tess-TOSS-ter-own) or, more simply, DHT. One of the functions of DHT is that it "hooks up" chemically with a specific protein receptor, moves to the nucleus of the cell, and subsequently becomes a powerful force in transmitting genetic information from prostate cells.[62] Higher concentrations of both DHT and proteins—called "growth factors"—that have been found in removed BPH tissue suggest that when DHT is transported to the nuclei of prostate cells, it sets off "a cascade of events" that results in the production of these proteins, which in turn stimulate tissue growth.[63]

Other researchers and urologists speculate that BPH may develop as a result of genetic programming. Instructions carried in the DNA of some prostate cells may cause them to "awaken" at a certain time and deliver signals to other cells that makes them more sensitive to hormones that influence growth.[64] Still other scientists believe that the nervous system of older men sends messages to tighten up the muscle tissue of the prostate.

A fourth possibility involves the increased production of the hormone estrogen, because men normally produce a certain amount of estrogen. Increased accumulation in the smooth muscle (stroma) of the prostate occurs as aging and decreased testosterone production occur. In contrast, DHT content does not follow an age-dependent decrease in the stroma, but does decrease with age in the epithelium of the prostate, leading to a tremendous increase with age of the estrogen/androgen ratio in the human prostate.

Could it be that a balanced androgen/estrogen synergism is necessary to maintain a normal human prostate?[65] According to the Internet home page for the National Institute of Diabetes and Digestive and Kidney Disease (NIDDK)—established by Congress in 1950 as one of the National Institutes of Health—animal studies suggest that higher amounts of estrogen may increase the activity of substances that make cells grow.[66]

One European urologist, George Debled, M.D., believes that the decreased level of testosterone, which raises the estrogen/testosterone ratio, is what causes problems in the muscles of the bladder and prostate. According to Dr. Michael Schachter, Dr. Debled gives his patients additional testosterone to relieve prostate problems and has even found a much lower incidence of prostate cancer than would be expected.[67] Unfortunately, Dr. Schachter gives us neither facts or figures, nor research studies that we can review. Many American doctors, believing that high levels of testosterone may result in prostate cancer, would be unlikely to advocate Dr. Debled's treatment.

WHY SOME MEN NEVER GET BPH

Several small groups of men have been identified who do not develop BPH or prostate cancer. Studying their characteristics has helped researchers understand more about what causes BPH and how it can be controlled.

The most well-known such group of men who do not develop BPH are those who've been castrated. For various reasons, they've had their testicles removed surgically—a century ago it was a common "cure" for BPH—or shrunk by taking female hormones such as estrogen. After castration, their bodies no longer produce testosterone.

In 1974, two independent groups described for the first time in separate reputable journals (*Science* and the *New England Journal of Medicine*) a small group of males who, although genetically male, at birth had external genitalia that were atypical of "normal" male babies.[68] They had normal male internal duct structures and normally differentiated testes. At puberty, with the increase in testosterone, their voices deepened and their penises enlarged.[69] Laboratory research indicated that these children had a genetically linked deficiency in 5-alpha-reductase, which you will remember is the enzyme that converts testosterone into the more active hormone dihydrotestosterone (DHT). In other words, these men were unable to metabolize testosterone into the more potent DHT.

Since those first studies, other men with the same genetic deficiency, which biochemical investigations have now localized to chromosome 2,[70] also have been identified. Biopsies of their prostate glands reveal only stroma cells, most likely associated with muscle tissue, and no epithelium.[71]

As these men mature, they develop a normal male libido and potency; however, their prostates remain small throughout adulthood. They have less body and facial hair than most men. They seldom have acne during adolescence; their hairline doesn't recede as they age; and they don't become bald.[72]

The scientists who studied the biology and genetic makeup of these men discovered that the substance 5-alpha-reductase plays an important role in normal male sexual differentiation and in controlling the development of secondary sexual characteristics at puberty. Their knowledge helped lead to the development of a model for predicting the long-term effects of using pharmaceuticals to inhibit the production of 5-alpha-reductase. This in turn has led to Merck Research Laboratories' development of Proscar—one of the leading pharmaceuticals now used to treat enlarged prostates.[73]

• • •

You may think that our discussion of BPH paints a complicated, unpleasant, and painful future for men to look forward to as they move through their lives. We *do* hope we've made it clear that BPH is not a condition men can take lightly, but we *do not* mean to depress you with prospects of a miserable and unremitting future filled with increasing pain and discomfort.

BPH is serious and, unfortunately, most doctors in the United States think it requires surgery or medication. However, a revolution is at hand, and *The Prostate Cure* is leading the charge. Today men want to learn more about their bodies and the options available to them. They want to feel empowered to make the right decisions about medications or surgery that may significantly effect the quality of their lives. As millions have discovered, questions about intimate and difficult issues like impotence and incontinence call for some of the most important decisions a man will ever make. They shouldn't be brusquely dictated by doctors, but rather carefully considered by their family members.

In the upcoming chapters, we'll analyze some of the standard approaches to treating BPH and uncover some recently developed treatments that have proven more effective—and less painful and less expensive—than surgery.

2

STANDARD NON-ORAL APPROACHES
TO TREATING BPH

How does a doctor determine that a man has BPH?

*

What are the treatments for BPH?

*

Is surgery absolutely necessary?

*

*What is the difference between a simple
and a radical prostatectomy?*

*

What are the newer surgical-like procedures?

*

*Does medical treatment for BPH always
require hospitalization?*

With this chapter, we begin a review of the non-oral options that men have had up to now for treatment of an enlarged prostate. We'll focus on the steps a doctor and patient will take to confirm the diagnosis of BPH and to rule out other possibilities. We continue by considering the first two of three options currently available for men with BPH: watchful waiting and surgery, which includes the newer surgical-like procedures.

MAKING THE BPH DIAGNOSIS

The first step in treating BPH is to ensure a correct diagnosis. Evaluation procedures include compiling a detailed medical history in order to identify other possible causes of urinary difficulties, or to pinpoint other ailments that may complicate treatment (more about the doctor's initial evaluation in Chapter 3).

Sometime during this first meeting/evaluation, the doctor will conduct a physical examination that includes a digital rectal exam (DRE). Either before or after the DRE, the doctor may order one or more laboratory tests, including a urinalysis and a blood test. Although the urinalysis does not directly contribute to the diagnosis of BPH, it helps the doctor rule out urinary tract infection (shown by the presence of a large number of white blood cells or by bacteria) and look for blood in the urine, which may indicate BPH, but can also warn of kidney or bladder disease. The blood tests will help rule out other disorders, and typically include a determination of PSA (prostate-specific antigen) and alkaline phosphatase levels (to screen for cancer), and a serum creatinine measurement to determine whether or not there are kidney complications.

In one study of the tests that 226 primary care physicians use in their diagnostic procedure, 66 percent reported routinely ordering tests to determine the serum creatinine level.[1] Other diagnostic procedures might include urodynamic measurements of urine flow and bladder pressure to help determine the degree of obstruction and the functioning of the bladder and urinary sphincters.

In some cases the doctor may suggest additional, specialized tests to be done another time, especially if you are a first-time patient. He may order a transrectal ultrasound, and/or rectal coil magnetic resonance imaging (MRI) in order to see the degree of obstruction in the prostate as well as any bladder changes that have been caused by the obstruction.

The doctor may also recommend a cystoscopy, an uncomfortable procedure in which he inserts a tube that contains a lens and a light system through the opening of the urethra, after a solution is sent into the urethra that numbs the inside of the penis. With the cystoscope, the doctor can determine the size of the gland and identify the location and degree of the obstruction of the urethra. The cystoscopic exam can also give an accurate measurement of the amount of residual urine in the bladder if the doctor has had the patient urinate immediately prior to the exam. As the cystoscope enters the bladder, any urine that remains inside comes out of the cystoscope and can be collected and measured. The more residual urine (especially if it exceeds 100 milliliters), the greater the need for surgical treatment.[2]

Fortunately, all of the diagnostic procedures discussed in the preceding two paragraphs can be accomplished on an outpatient basis. Their names probably sound worse than the actual techniques, but they are expensive and most likely will not be routine tests.

HOW IS BPH TREATED?

Evaluation of the treatment options for the man with BPH include considering not only the severity of the symptoms—although that may be the impetus to see the doctor—but also the type of treatment appropriate for a particular patient. This, in turn, is influenced by the risk entailed, the advantages/disadvantages in any procedure or medication chosen, and the health-related quality of life with and without treatment.

Both direct considerations (costs of diagnosis, management, treatment, and posttreatment monitoring) and indirect considerations (loss of work time, negative impact on well-being) should also be taken into account.[3] Sometimes the existence of other health problems will necessarily influence the decision.

Natural history studies now show that progression of BPH to severe symptoms is rare.[4] As already noted in Chapter 1, almost all men will develop enlarged prostates as a natural consequence of aging, yet clinical symptoms develop in only 50 percent of patients with a palpably enlarged prostate gland.[5]

Although there are several medical options that are under investigation—and more will undoubtedly will be introduced over the next decade—at present there are three major ways that BPH is treated:

- *Watchful waiting*
- *Surgery*
- *Medications*

Watchful waiting is usually recommended for men with mild symptoms that have little or no impact on the activities of their daily life. For men with moderate-to-severe symptoms, a variety of medical and pharmaceutical therapies are available. Surgical options have been expanded in the last two decades to include new minimally invasive procedures, which vastly improve upon the open prostatectomy, the standard procedure early in the century.

Before we review these therapies in detail, let's consider briefly a 1996 observational study conducted by several researchers associated with the Harvard School of Public Health to evaluate the effectiveness of the three modes of treatment for BPH. This study included a total of 1,459 men, aged 48 to 84 years, who were diagnosed in 1994 by physicians for the first time as having BPH and who had not received treatment. During a one-year follow-up, 1,064 (72.9 percent) of the men remained on no treatment (watchful waiting); 156 (10.7 percent) were treated with a medication called finasteride (more about that in Chapter 3); 198 (13.6 percent) were treated with an alpha-blocker medication (see Chapter 3, "Alpha-adrenergic Blockers"); while the smallest number (41, or 2.8 percent) underwent

> *Researcher M. J. Barry estimates that if current rates of surgery persist for BPH, the average 40-year-old man in the United States will have a 30 to 40 percent chance of undergoing a prostatectomy if he survives to age 80.*[6]

prostatectomies. Men who underwent the surgery reported the biggest improvements in lower urinary tract symptoms.[7]

Yet an earlier study shows that patients with very mild symptoms do not benefit from surgery for BPH.[8] Men with moderate symptoms of BPH are considered by some to be the best candidates for pharmaceutical treatment, while surgery is usually indicated for patients with severe symptoms.[9]

In 1995, H. L. Holtgrewe, chairman of a committee that was writing on the economics of BPH, reported the following individual direct costs associated with various treatments for BPH to a group of doctors attending the Third International Conference on BPH:[10]

Primary Treatment Modality	*Cost of Primary Treatment and 1-Year Follow-up*	*Cost of Second Year of Follow-up*
Watchful waiting	$ 1,162	$640
Finasteride	$ 1,326	$788
Alpha-adrenergic Blocker	$ 1,395	$845
TURP (simple prostatectomy)	$ 8,606	$360
Open prostatectomy	$12,788	$ 69

These figures do not include indirect costs such as the patient's lost wages and absence from work. Of course, the numbers have certainly increased as medical costs have soared since 1995, and, as you will see in this chapter, more medical options are being developed all the time. So, while these figures are already out of date, they do give some sense of cost comparison between the medical options available at the time.

With these figures in mind, and in spite of the findings of the Harvard School of Public Health's 1996 study and the predictions of Dr. Barry, we will show in Chapter 3 and throughout the remainder of the book that there *are* additional things a man with BPH can do, which his doctor likely will not suggest, that have worked for some men. These include the addition of Cernitin to your diet, the possible inclusion of herb and vitamin supplements, and lifestyle changes.

WATCHFUL WAITING

From a physician's viewpoint, watchful waiting (as its name implies) means no active treatment, but periodic examinations to evaluate progression of BPH. It is appropriate for many men, particularly those who are asymptomatic or have only mild symptoms, and whose enlarged prostate was likely found through the digital rectal examination.

The natural history of untreated BPH is poorly documented in the literature. Both the symptoms and the severity of obstruction can fluctuate considerably over time. Some studies have shown that a significant proportion of men with moderate BPH symptoms (between 50 and 75 percent) experienced either stabilization or improvement of their symptoms in the absence of any therapeutic intervention.[11]

More recent studies show that about 30 percent of men with BPH will experience little or no change in symptoms with watchful waiting. For unknown reasons, a small number (about 15 percent) actually improve with time; however, some 56 percent of men are likely to experience a worsening of their symptoms.[12]

A study conducted with 40 Singapore men, for instance, found that it does not always follow that the degree to which patients are "bothered" is analogous to symptom severity and that it should, therefore, be considered independently in treatment-related decision making.[13]

A British survey of 1,271 men in 12 countries who had lower urinary tract symptoms concluded that voiding symptoms were the most prevalent and correlated with age, whereas the most bothersome—storage symptoms, including incontinence—were relatively unrelated to age.[14]

Certainly it appears that the decision to select watchful waiting as a "treatment" choice depends not only on the physical discomfort of a man's symptoms and his restriction in activities, but also on other quality-of-life considerations such as the discomfort level and lifestyle restrictions, and how worrisome the condition is for the man involved.[15]

WHEN SURGERY BECOMES NECESSARY

Only 20 percent of patients with symptomatic BPH undergo surgical treatment because of complications of BPH, such as deterioration of kidney function related to chronic retention of urine, recurrent or chronic urinary tract infections, recurrent episodes of urinary retention, bladder stones, and episodes of blood in the urine.[16] Whether a man needs to have surgery for his BPH depends, therefore, on the severity of the urethral obstruction, the degree of pain and discomfort he experiences, and whether surgery is the only option for relieving it.

As indicated in Chapter 1, the prostate enlarges over time, and the new growth initially tends to extend inward in the middle lobe of the prostate toward the prostatic urethra, and then outward toward the dense and fibrous shell of the outside of the prostate gland. Tissue that has grown outward into the two lateral lobes can be felt during a digital rectal examination as an enlarged prostate—but it is the inward, rather than the outward, growth that brings about those frustrating symptoms associated with BPH described in Chapter 1. The enlarging middle lobe, which causes all the troubling symptoms, can never be felt during a digital rectal exam.

Where the enlarging tissue meets the normal and true prostate tissue is called the "surgical capsule." During surgery for BPH, the new growth of BPH tissue—all the tissue that lies within the surgical capsule—is what is removed, leaving behind only the true prostate tissue.[17]

Once you get into considering surgical treatments, or prostatectomies, for BPH, you enter a world populated by bewildering acronyms. Actually the term "prostatectomy" as applied to BPH is a misnomer, since by definition prostatectomy means removal of the prostate. In procedures for BPH, only the part of the prostate that is causing obstruction is removed. In order to distinguish it from a "radical prostatectomy" (when the entire gland is removed, as in cancer surgery), surgery for BPH is also known as a "simple prostatectomy," or TURP. Of the 400,000 prostatectomies performed annually in the United States, more than 90 percent[18] are TURPs, at a cost that exceeds $1 billion.[19] Prostatectomy is the second leading cost of Medicare reimbursement (behind cataract extraction) in men age 65 or older.[20]

While most doctors believe that a simple prostatectomy offers the best and fastest chance for improving BPH, this treatment may not totally alleviate the symptoms of discomfort. For instance, surgery may remove the obstruction, but symptoms may persist due to bladder abnormalities.[21] Surgery is also associated with the greatest number of long-term complications, including impotence, incontinence, and retrograde ejaculation (ejaculation of semen into the bladder rather than through the penis). Ten percent of the men electing to have a simple prostatectomy require a second surgery after five years due to continued prostate growth or a urethral stricture (scarring or narrowing) resulting from the initial surgery.[22] A major problem with all the varieties of simple prostatectomies that we discuss in the remainder of this chapter is that they leave behind much of the prostate gland, so it is still possible for prostate problems—including BPH—to develop again.

As you will see throughout this book, a variety of new options is making surgery less necessary. Treatment for BPH has changed drastically within the past three years, and will likely continue to change in the future.

TRANSURETHRAL RESECTION OF THE PROSTATE (TURP)

The "gold standard" against which all other treatments for BPH are measured is a transurethral prostatectomy or transurethral resection of the prostate, commonly referred to as TURP, and, more flippantly, as the "Roto-Rooter" of prostatectomies. Although TURP has been the surgical treatment of choice for BPH for the past 50 years, and the one against which all newer techniques are compared, 20 percent of patients experience clinically significant adverse reactions following the surgery,[23] and between 5 percent[24] and 15 percent[25] require a second operation after two years of follow-up.

TURP involves removing those portions of the prostate that are obstructing the urethra by inserting an instrument called a resecto-

> *An estimate based on medical insurance claims*
> *indicates that one in five men will undergo a*
> *second TURP operation due to failure of the*
> *original surgery to stop prostate growth.*[26]

scope through the urethra into the bladder. It uses a telescopic hot wire loop that emits a high-frequency electrical current to cut like an electric knife through the prostate gland, working outward until the surgical capsule is reached. The pieces of tissue that are cut away, called "chips," are carried by irrigating fluid into the bladder and then flushed out through the resectoscope. Samples of tissue are sent to a laboratory to be examined for prostate cancer. TURP is the operation of choice for small and moderate growths of BPH, but not for patients with massive BPH,[27] since it is technically difficult to do in such cases.

TURP is major "surgery." Although no incision is made, general or spinal anesthesia is required. It is a delicate procedure, requires a skilled surgeon, and can take anywhere from 30 to 90 minutes to complete. Hospitalization lasts from two to five days (a tube or catheter is inserted in the bladder for the first two to three days), after which a man can expect to spend two to four weeks at home recovering.

Significant side effects associated with TURP include temporary bleeding, the chance of urinary or other infection (as with any surgery), retrograde ejaculation (occurring in 70 to 75 percent of patients),[28] temporary urinary retention after removal of the catheter, impotence (occurring in 5 to 10 percent of cases), and incontinence (in 2 to 4 percent of cases), not to mention cardiac risk due to anesthesia.[29] In addition, anywhere from 2 to 10 percent of patients require blood transfusions.[30] Late postoperative complications include urethral stricture (abnormal narrowing or constriction) and contractures of the bladder neck.[31]

Medical studies differ with regard to exact statistics on impotence caused by the surgery, because apparently many men may be impotent and undiagnosed before TURP is performed. In a review of the literature, Dr. Teuvo Tammela, a urologist associated with Tampere University Hospital in Tampere, Finland, cited a 1995 study that suggested that there were virtually no new cases of impotence or incontinence after TURP.[32]

When doctors at Kaiser Permanente Medical Center in Oakland reviewed the records of 4,708 patients who had undergone TURP from 1976 to 1984, and compared them to an age-matched group of 4,708 randomly selected members of the program not undergoing surgery, the relative risk of death for surgery versus no surgery was determined to be less than 1 percent (0.88). When examined by five-year age-group intervals, the relative risk ranged from 0.77 to 0.95 percent.[33]

TRANSURETHRAL INCISION OF THE PROSTATE (TUIP)

An alternative to TURP, transurethral incision of the prostate (TUIP) is a more limited surgical procedure that can sometimes be used for men with relatively small prostate enlargement. Although TUIP has a lower risk of operative complications, it is, unfortunately, not appropriate for all men with BPH.

First used in the United States in the early 1970s, TUIP is also done with an instrument that is passed through the urethra, so no skin incision is made. The surgeon makes one or two deep cuts (incisions) with a knife or laser along the entire prostate to split it. The procedure allows the circular muscle fibers running around the prostate to spring open. A TUIP increases urinary flow by opening the prostatic urethra. No attempt is made to remove any obstructing prostate tissue.

Men who elect to have TUIPs experience a lower incidence of ejaculation abnormalities, plus their hospital stays and recovery times are shorter. In many cases, TUIP is performed under local anesthesia on an outpatient basis. It is not yet clear whether the curative effects of TUIP are as lasting as those of TURP. About 1 to 2 percent of men who have either TURP or TUIP require repeat surgery.[34]

TRANSURETHRAL MICROWAVE THERMOTHERAPY (TUMT)

Transurethral microwave thermotherapy, or TUMT, is considered a minimally invasive procedure because it can be carried out in a single session, without the use of general or regional anesthesia, in an office-based or outpatient setting. It utilizes a microwave probe (approved by the FDA in 1996) placed into the prostatic channel. The probe heats prostate tissue to temperatures above 50 degrees C, destroying the tissue and shrinking the gland.

Newer microwave machines use a catheter that cools the lining of the prostatic urethra while heating the prostate tissue, resulting in less irritation during healing. The newer instruments can also better control delivery of microwave energy and heat level, and their use is commonly known as high-energy transurethral microwave thermotherapy (HE-TUMT). For men with more severe bladder outlet obstruction, the higher-energy treatment protocols seem to work better.[35]

In lower-energy TUMT, analgesia and pain medication are often not required and the patient's perception of discomfort is described as varying from a "mild feeling of perineal discomfort and warmth to moderate urgency during the procedure." Approximately 20 to 25 percent of patients will experience urinary retention for an average of seven days, necessitating the use of a catheter.[36] With the high-energy treatment, pain medication is necessary for patient comfort, and urinary retention is expected.

Possible side effects associated with TUMT, as reported in medical literature, include temporary discomfort during the treatment, bleeding, and the possibility of infection. It has a lower risk of impotence and incontinence than TURP. While TUMT did not alter hormone levels, 21 patients who reported favorable response to the treatment after one year had significantly lower outset levels of free testosterone than did 27 nonresponders. This finding suggests the possibility that the androgen-sensitive tissue in men with a higher degree of androgen stimulation may be more resistant to treatment regimes based on partial destruction (as in TUMT).[37]

A 1997 review by Dutch doctors of all the data available from the medical literature showed unequivocal support for the efficacy and safety of TUMT for treatment of symptomatic BPH, with significant improvement in objective and subjective parameters.[38] In studies to date, however, 20 to 25 percent of patients who have been treated with TUMT failed to respond.[39]

Another review of the medical literature regarding various procedures for BPH conducted by doctors from the Palo Alto Veterans Administration Hospital and at the Stanford University School of Medicine, discovered that, for a hypothetical 70-year-old potent man with moderate symptoms of BPH, TUMT would provide more quality-of-life months at a cheaper overall cost than would TURP. These researchers conclude that TUMT just might be the new "gold standard" for treatment of BPH.[40]

A British study compared the effects of TUMT with TURP by using two groups of 30 patients each, who were technically suitable for either form of treatment, and randomly selecting which procedure they would undergo. The variables compared before and after the procedures were the symptom score of the American Urological Association (AUA), maximum urinary flow rate, postvoid residual urine volume, voiding pressure and prostatic volume (determined by ultrasonography), plus complications. After TURP, all variables improved clinically, while after TUMT the AUA symptoms improved both clinically and statistically; however, none of the objective variables improved.[41]

Another double-blind study conducted by some of the same doctors found similar lack of improvement in the same objective variables, but found that at six months AUA symptoms (the subjective variable) were rated as improved at about the same level in a group of patients who underwent a standard TUMT and those who underwent a "simulated" TUMT.[42] An untreated control group showed neither clinically relevant deterioration nor improvement.[43]

In the first study, ejaculation failure occurred in 4 of 18 sexually active men after TUMT. The doctors conducting that study indicate that TUMT did not alleviate obstruction in patients with BPH and that patients electing this procedure should be informed of the possibility of ejaculatory dysfunction.[44]

A study conducted at the University Hospital at Nijmegen in The Netherlands investigated the use of HE-TUMT in an outpatient setting on a series of 301 patients between 45 and 89 years of age. Because no research was available at the time on the long-term efficacy of HE-TUMT, this study was the first to contain data from a large patient group over such a lengthy follow-up time. At the two-year follow-up, the procedure resulted in a good outcome in 93 percent of patients, with an objective improvement rate of 42 percent and a subjective improvement rate of 65 percent.[45]

Members of the same team of Dutch doctors compared the outcome of TURP and HE-TUMT for 52 BPH patients (21 treated with TURP, 31 with HE-TUMT) during a one-year follow-up period.

Symptomatic improvement was 78 percent in the TURP group compared with 68 percent in the HE-TURP group. Improvements in free flow rate were 100 percent for the TURP men and 69 percent for those in the thermotherapy group. No serious complications occurred in either group, while one patient in each group required repeat treatment.[46]

In the past six years, TUMT has introduced and helped define the concept of "minimally invasive therapy" for BPH. As improvements in technology occur, further research using TUMT is being directed toward identifying more exact criteria for selecting men who will benefit from the procedure and in determining the optimal thermal dose that will maintain safe treatment while resulting in significant improvement and minimum morbidity.[47]

While many reports are beginning to establish the effectiveness and safety of TUMT, it is still difficult to predict the response to TUMT on an individual basis. Because it is a relatively new procedure, the long-term benefits and risks of TUMT are as yet unknown, and that is also true for all of the procedures that follow.

TRANSURETHRAL NEEDLE ABLATION (TUNA)

Any thermotherapy for BPH is based on the principle that heating prostate tissue—or any human tissue for that matter—above certain temperatures (usually 40–50 degrees C) will cause the tissue to die.

Transurethral needle ablation (TUNA) of the prostate involves using a catheter with a fiberoptic system inside it that is inserted in the urethra. With the TUNA procedure, tiny needles are inserted sequentially through the tip of the catheter into various sectors of the prostate; then low-energy radio waves delivered by the needles heat the water molecules in the prostate tissue to more than 100 degrees C. Insulating sheaths protect the urethra from heat damage. Absorption of the dead tissue occurs during the ensuing eight weeks. (Patients often experience little improvement in voiding symptoms for the first two to three weeks, before tissue absorption begins and a large enough channel develops around the urethra to decrease constriction and enable urine to flow through the urethra comfortably.)

TUNA requires only a local anesthetic and is done on an outpatient basis. Many urologists leave a catheter in place for three days; others send the patent home without a catheter provided he can void satisfactorily following the procedure. Antibiotic therapy is required before the surgery and for at least 48 hours following catheter removal. After the catheter is removed, patients may experience a weak stream and worse voiding symptoms for two to four days until the prostatic swelling has subsided. There may be no improvement in voiding symptoms for two to six weeks following the procedure and although symptoms progressively improve for eight to 10 weeks after the procedure, full improvement may take as long as three months.[48]

Most patients have blood in their urine for 12 to 14 hours after the procedure. Urinary retention occurs in about 20 percent of patients not catheterized postoperatively. Postoperative urinary tract infections are rare, occurring in only about 1 percent of patients, and neither incontinence nor impotence after the TUNA procedure has been reported in any study.[49] Patients electing to have laser ablation or any form of thermotherapy should be aware that there can be no laboratory examination of prostate tissue to determine the presence of cancer.[50]

TUNA may very well be the treatment of choice for men with small to moderate-sized prostate enlargement and for elderly or other patients who are at poor risk for TURP or a prostatectomy. Although TUNA can be utilized for some patients with large prostates, it may require six or seven treatments performed at one-centimeter levels along the lateral lobe of the prostate.[51] In studies employing TUNA, the procedure appears to allow more precise targeting of prostate tissue and offer less risk of damaging surrounding organs.

A study conducted at Sheba Medical Center in Tel-Hashomer, Israel, followed 76 TUNA patients from five centers. Sixty-eight patients were available for follow-up after one year. The procedure produced significant improvements in the International Prostate Symptom Score (IPPS), urinary flow rate, and quality-of-life considerations.[52]

When 120 men with urinary obstruction due to BPH were treated with TUNA at the Predabissi Hospital in Milan, Italy, overall the patients showed a decrease in irritative symptoms, as measured by the IPPS, and an increase in peak flow rate which continued upon reevaluation at 12 and 18 months. When 72 of the men in the study were reevaluated at one year, 30 (41.7 percent) had no obstruction, 30 had "equivocal" results (not specified), while 12 (16.6 percent) still had obstruction. The researchers conclude that TUNA produces better results in patients with moderate to severe irritative symptoms and minimal obstruction (determined by pressure/flow studies).[53]

Drs. Simeon Margolis and H. Ballentine Carter, authors of the 1997 *Johns Hopkins White Paper on Prostate Disorders,* cite information from the first U.S. study to examine the results of TUNA. The procedure was performed on 12 BPH patients, age 56 to 76, who were then examined periodically during the next six months. There was an overall 61 percent reduction in the American Urology Association (AUA) index scores, and 70 percent higher scores on a quality-of-life test. Side effects were considered minor (12 had mild pain or difficulty urinating for one to seven days; five had urinary retention for one to four days). One patient experienced retrograde ejaculation.[54]

HIGH-INTENSITY FOCUSED ULTRASOUND (HIFU)

Reports are beginning to show up in the medical literature on the use of HIFU, high-intensity focused ultrasound, which uses a probe placed in the rectum to selectively blast BPH tissue and form cavities in the prostate. Ultrasound energy can be focused with such "exquisite precision" that even tissue a fraction of an inch away from the target area is not heated or damaged, sparing surrounding tissue. However, the high temperature employed requires either spinal or local anesthesia during the procedure for comfort.[55]

In 1997, a group of doctors in Dublin, Ireland, assessed the results of HIFU in clinical trials of 13 patients, including objective evaluations of prostate size and post-void residual urine volume, plus subjective satisfaction. Assessments were conducted at regular intervals for two years following the procedure. Subjective symptoms, as measured by the International Prostate Symptom Score, decreased considerably, from an average of 23 before treatment to 5 after one year and 7 after two years. Both the size of the prostate and the amount of post-void residual volume decreased. Although there was an initial improvement in flow rates, these subsequently declined. The doctors conclude that HIFU should not be used as an alternative to more well-established treatment modalities until it has been assessed more fully in randomized trials.[56]

In a Canadian hospital in Vancouver, 25 patients were treated with HIFU and evaluated before and after one treatment, using the American Urological Association (AUA) symptom score, peak urinary flow rate, and a quality-of-life score. Five patients with large glands were withdrawn because the failure rate was high. The remaining 20 patients showed improvements in the AUA symptom scores, urinary flow rate, and quality-of-life scores.[57]

LASER PROSTATECTOMIES

In the laser prostatectomy procedure, a surgeon passes a laser fiber into the prostatic channel and then destroys obstructing portions of the prostate by heating it up. During a laser prostatectomy, BPH tissue is not removed. Rather, space is created around the urethra when the heated tissue dies, sloughs away into the urine, or is absorbed back into the body.[58]

One common type of laser prostatectomy is known as transurethral ultrasound-guided laser-induced prostatectomy (TULIP). TULIP features a probe containing an optical laser fiber and paired ultrasound transducers. The ultrasound scanner gives the surgeon a "picture" of the areas the laser will target, thus providing greater accuracy. The probe is passed inside a balloon, which is inflated in the prostatic urethra. This permits the transmission of ultrasound and laser energy while, at the same time, holding the prostate tissue in place. The balloon compresses the prostatic tissue, making it more uniform, and also decreases the blood supply.[59]

Patients who undergo laser prostatectomy do not require hospitalization, since there is no postoperative bleeding, and the procedure requires only regional or local anesthesia.[60] Critics of TULIP say that its reliance on state-of-the-art equipment makes the procedure too technical and expensive for use in many medical centers.[61]

Two other techniques using lasers are transurethral laser vaporization (TUVP) and visual laser ablation of the prostate (VLAP). High instantaneous heat is created with TUVP in order to steam away, or vaporize the tissue. VLAP employs a lower level of laser energy to heat up the tissue just enough to dry it out, so it can shrink and slough away with time. VLAP requires multiple treatments if the prostate is large, while TUVP can remove more tissue in one treatment.

Doctors at the Veterans General Hospital in Taipei, Taiwan, conducted a study of 30 men ranging in age from 60 to 83, who were treated with TUVP for symptomatic BPH. At three months after surgery, the procedure had increased urine flow and decreased other American Urological Association symptom scores. The doctors suggest, however, that a cautious attitude be adopted toward its use, in view of the possibility of late complications. Three of the patients (10 percent) developed bladder neck contracture. Of the 24 patients who were sexually potent before the operation, three (12.5 percent) became impotent.[62]

VLAP was first performed in Australia in 1991.[63] In the VLAP procedure, a laser is inserted through a cystoscope into the urethra to the area of the prostate. Heat from the laser kills the excess tissue, which then sloughs into the urine or is absorbed by the body. The procedure requires 15 to 60 minutes and can be performed with intravenous sedation.[64]

Compared to TURP, the advantages of VLAP are minimal bleeding, reduced surgical time, and shorter hospitalization stay. Yet, all laser procedures seem to produce a greater amount of swelling around the prostate channel (similar to the way tissue swells around a burn) for some 3 to 10 days, which requires a catheter for bladder drainage. Some men experience urinary frequency for a few weeks and painful irritation while the prostatic channel is healing. VLAP also draws fire from urologists who say that its low-tech approach yields satisfactory results only when used by expert surgeons.[65]

Doctors at the Furuya Hospital in Kitami, Japan, have employed transurethral balloon laser thermotherapy (TUBAL-T) with 12 patients who were considered poor candidates for prostatectomy (i.e., were at high risk for surgery). The ages of the men ranged from 66 to 93 years, with an average age of 78.9 years. The technique involved radiating the prostatic tissue from 40 to 54 minutes (average 45.2 minutes) with a laser balloon placed in the prostatic urethra. Successful resumption of long-term spontaneous voiding was achieved for nine of the 12 men, with the longest being 34 months.[66]

ONCE-POPULAR, SELDOM-USED PROCEDURES

We include here mention of a couple of once-common procedures for treating BPH, because men consulting the most popular books on BPH will still find them listed, although they are now considered out-of-date by most urologists.

OPEN SURGERY

In the few cases where a transurethral procedure cannot be used, open surgery, which requires an external incision in the lower abdomen, may be used. Applicable situations include cases where the gland is greatly enlarged, where there are complicating factors, or where the bladder has been damaged and needs to be repaired. Today the procedure is likely to be needed in only 2 to 3 percent of men with BPH.[67]

In the past, open surgery for BPH was carried out either through an incision in the perineum (the area between the scrotum and the rectum) in a procedure called a perineal prostatectomy, or through a lower abdominal incision. Due to the higher risk of injury to surrounding organs, perineal prostatectomies have largely been abandoned.[68]

BALLOON DILATION

Transurethral dilation of the prostate gland (balloon dilation) became quite common during the 1980s and is still included in many books

> Approximately 80 percent of patients who undergo balloon dilation will require further treatment within the next four years.[69] Because of this, many doctors no longer use balloon dilation.

of that era written about the prostate. In this procedure, which employs a local anesthetic, a catheter is used to place an uninflated balloon in the portion of the urethra that lies within the prostate. The balloon is then inflated to stretch the urethra and reduce the amount of obstruction. Most useful in patients with relative small prostates, improvement tends to diminish with time and often does not last for more than a year.[70]

STILL-DEVELOPING TECHNIQUES AND INNOVATIONS

New techniques beyond the various kinds of prostatectomies and techniques presented in this chapter are being created and tested. By the time this book is in print, there will likely be at least one more, if not several, and certainly there will be several more within the next five years, say urologists J. B. Hollander and A. C. Diokno.[71]

Internet website pages offer good up-to-date information on the latest clinical trials or newest innovations for treating BPH. For instance, it was from the website of the Columbia-Presbyterian Prostate Center in New York that we learned that Doctors Steven Kaplan and Alexis Te, surgeons at the Center, have pioneered a new electrosurgical technique called electrovaporization of the prostate, which, as its name implies, employs electrical energy to vaporize the prostate gland.[72]

Still in clinical trials, it involves the use of a specially designed, grooved rollerball electrode that heats the tissues of the prostate gland until they turn into steam, which are then washed away by a constant flow of water. As the electrode moves to fresh tissue, that too is removed. The resulting pathway does not bleed because it is coagulated and sealed by the electrically heated rolling action of the electrode. Several types of anesthesia can be used, including general, regional, and intravenous sedation. Of the initial 25 patients on which the surgery was performed, three (12 percent) had slight blood in the urine, which disappeared within three weeks, and some patients experienced a postoperative side effect of painful, irritative urination.[73] Apparently as the technique is perfected, and the number of persons on whom it is used increases, the postoperative irritative symptom has decreased.

When doctors at the University Hospital of Wales in Cardiff employed the technique on 116 patients over a 10-month period, they followed up the patients every four months during the first postoperative year. Symptom scores improved by 67 percent, residual volumes improved by 72 percent, and urine flow rates increased from 8.5 milliliters per second before treatment to 10.5 at the first four-month review. The procedure had an average operative time of

If the new electrovaporization technique continues to be successful—and it seems likely that it will— its major potential advantages over TURP will be reduced cost, fewer side effects, less bleeding during surgery, shorter catheterization time (24 hours) and hospital stay, and a more rapid convalescence time.

35 minutes, with a range of 20 to 65 minutes, and no patients required a blood transfusion. Most patients had their catheters removed within 24 hours and were discharged on the second day after treatment.[74]

Another technique, which has been around longer but has yet to receive FDA approval (although it is used in Great Britain and the Scandinavian countries), involves opening blocked urinary passages by placing plastic or wire devices shaped like small springs or coils, called stents, in a man's urethra to stretch the channel and keep it open. Their positioning takes about 20 minutes and requires only a local anesthesia. Since the major problem with stents relates to the irritation and debris that form on the stent, resulting in a higher incidence of urinary tract infections, they are used conservatively for patients who medically cannot tolerate a surgical procedure that requires a greater level of anesthesia. Removal of the device is required in at least 10 percent of patients within the first year because of persistent irritation, treatment failure, or encrustation with urinary tract infection.[75] Little is known about their long-term effects.

Doctors at the Kouseiren Kamo Hospital in Japan utilized stents with seven patients ranging in age from 68 to 86 years who had experienced acute urinary retention due to BPH. During the one-year follow-up period, all of the patients had satisfactory voiding with no complication or renal dysfunction. The Japanese doctors suggest that stents are a good alternative to an indwelling catheter for patients awaiting prostatic surgery and for those who, as indicated above, are either poor candidates for prostatectomy or are unwilling to undergo that procedure.[78]

•   •   •

Daunting as these medical procedures may seem to you, we want to remind you, once again, that they aren't the only options. So settle back and put surgery out of your mind for now as you consider more appealing possibilities.

In Chapter 3 we take a look at another medical option that is becoming more common and acceptable as the treatment of choice: medication. And we will also consider the effects of some of the more well-known herbal preparations on BPH symptoms.

Finally, in Chapter 4 we will present compelling scientific evidence regarding Cernitin, the safe, natural supplement that has proven time and again to be effective at shrinking enlarged prostates. We're certain that by the time you've finished *The Prostate Cure,* you will have a good idea of what products or procedures are available to you.

3

ALTERNATIVES TO SURGERY

What nonsurgical options are available for treating BPH?

*

What medicines are available for BPH?

*

What are the side effects of these medicines and how long must a man take them?

*

Are herbs having any effect on treating BPH?

*

What herbs are men using?

For men who choose not to have a prostatectomy, who don't require other surgical interventions, or whose additional health problems don't allow them to consider surgery, several nonsurgical medical therapies are available. Pharmacotherapy, or the use of medications, is rapidly becoming a popular alternative to surgery for BPH, especially in foreign countries.

PRESCRIBING DRUGS FOR BPH

Several prescription drugs are already in use for the treatment of BPH. Accompanying their entrance into the treatment arena is

In the United States, Medicare has shown a drop of more than 40 percent in the number of TURPs performed between 1987 and 1994, in spite of the increased number of men enrolled. Whether the actual decision was due to personal or insurance economics, or to a preference for doctor/patient alternatives to surgery, is unknown.[1]

extensive debate in the medical community about questions such as whether the drugs work at all, and if they do, which ones work better, and whether they should be combined for more effectiveness. The controversies arise largely out of criticisms about differences in the population of men selected for various studies, a factor which can considerably affect the "success" of the various drugs used in the studies, and which also makes comparison across studies difficult.

There is no doubt, however, that medications are having an impact on the type of health care men receive for BPH. One review of the usage and costs for BPH health care in Sweden from 1987 to 1994 indicated that TURP surgery decreased markedly after the introduction of medications, and that the use of TUMT procedures also decreased once medications were introduced. Drug sales showed that the number of men receiving drug treatment was greater than the annual number of men receiving TURP operations and TUMT procedures combined. Total costs of health care for BPH showed a slight decrease, due mainly to the decreasing numbers of TURP operations.[2]

When a nationwide survey of a random sample of 394 American urologists was conducted in 1995, 67 percent (264 doctors) responded and indicated that they had seen an average of 240 BPH patients during the preceding 12 months. The doctors had performed a median of 25 transurethral prostatectomies (TURPs), but few other operations for BPH. They had prescribed alpha-blockers for 70 patients and finasteride for 15. Clearly, where possible, watchful waiting and medications were the treatments of choice.[3]

ALPHA-ADRENERGIC BLOCKERS

Hytrin is the brand name of a systemic drug called terazosin (ter-AY-zoe-sin), which has been used to treat high blood pressure since 1987. The Food and Drug Administration (FDA) approved its use to treat BPH in 1993.

Hytrin is a long-acting, highly selective alpha-adrenergic blocking agent. It works by relaxing the smooth muscles in the prostate and the opening of the bladder. For many men, the urinary channel passage then opens enough to increase the flow of urine and also to decrease such symptoms as the need to urinate and a weak stream. In no way does it help shrink the prostate, however, which may continue to grow, resulting, ultimately, in the symptoms becoming worse over time. So, even though Hytrin may lessen some of the symptoms over a period of time as long as six weeks, surgery may still be needed in the future.

One of the major studies used to determine the effectiveness of Hytrin was a one-year clinical trial conducted by the University

Terazosin has the advantage of possessing a longer half-life than other alpha blockers, permitting once-daily administration.

of Texas Southwestern Medical Center at 15 academic medical centers and 141 private urology practices. Called the Hytrin Community Assessment Trial, the program enrolled a total of 1,084 men at least 55 years old who were experiencing moderate to severe symptoms of BPH. The men began by taking 1 mg of Hytrin daily for 3 days (to determine their tolerance for the drug), followed by 2 mg daily for 15 days. If a man failed to achieve a 35 percent or greater improvement in symptoms, he was titrated stepwise to a 5 or 10 mg dosage. Treatment results were objective, according to symptom scores as determined by the American Urological Association (AUA) symptom index, and subjective according to a "bother score."

AUA symptom scores improved by a statistically significant amount: 37.8 percent during use of Hytrin compared to only 18.4 percent during placebo treatment. Peak urinary flow rate also improved at a statistically significant level. Treatment failure occurred in 11.2 percent of the Hytrin-treated and 25.4 percent of the placebo-treated patients. Withdrawal from the study due to adverse events occurred in 19.7 percent of the Hytrin-treated patients and in 15.2 percent of the patients taking the placebo.[4]

Doctors have recommended that the dosage of Hytrin be gradually titrated from 1 mg to 2 mg, 5 mg, and, finally, if necessary to

Many studies show that persons using alpha-adrenergic blockers can maintain their improvements in both symptoms and flow rates for up to three years, and sometimes longer. For persons with high blood pressure, another advantage may be the successful treatment of two problems simultaneously.

10 mg until the dose with the best efficacy is reached. Controversy exists, however, regarding when to take the daily doses. One of Hytrin's most common side effects is dizziness or vertigo, due to the lowering of blood pressure. It occurs in 7.2 to 15.6 percent of patients.[5] Some physicians recommend that the dose be taken in the evening or at bedtime to avoid the dizziness that occurs upon standing (called postural hypotension) and other blood pressure-related side effects; however, it has also been shown that morning administration is as well tolerated by some patients.[6]

Other side effects can include chest pain, lightheadedness when rising from a lying or sitting position (1.9 to 3.9 percent of patients), sudden fainting, weakness, fatigue, and drowsiness (3.6 to 8 percent of patients), a fast, irregular, or pounding heartbeat (0.9 to 1.6 percent), shortness of breath, nasal congestion, and swelling of the feet or lower legs, and impotence (1.0 to 1.6 percent of patients).[7]

Other alpha-adrenergic blockers that work on the same principle as Hytrin include Cardura (doxazosin), with side effects of dizziness, drowsiness, and headaches;[8] and shorter-acting drugs such as Minipress (prazosin) and Xatral (alfuzosin). Minipress must be taken two to three times a day and may, like Cardura, cause dizziness and headaches.

A three-month, double-blind, placebo-controlled study involved 67 patients who received 4 mg of doxazosin daily and 68 patients who received a placebo. Patients treated with doxazosin experienced a statistically significant improvement in frequency (44 percent versus 27 percent), nocturia (39 percent versus 19 percent), urgency (60 percent versus 38 percent) and premicturition delay (56 percent versus 26 percent). The mean urinary flow rate also improved significantly for the treatment group compared to the placebo group.[9]

In contrast to other alpha-blockers, tamsulosin (brand name Flomax), which also needs to be taken only once daily, has no significant effect on blood pressure.[10] It is available in a modified release formulation, which enables men to take it once daily. In an American study, the adverse side effects that occurred significantly more often with tamsulosin than with a placebo were abnormal ejaculation and rhinitis (inflammation of the mucous membrane of the nose).[11]

ENZYME INHIBITORS

Proscar is the brand name of a form of finasteride (fi-NAS-teer-ide) used in the United States and Canada. It is an enzyme inhibitor. Specifically it blocks the enzyme called 5-alpha-reductase, which a man's body requires in order to change testosterone into dihydrotestosterone (DHT), the active androgenic metabolite in the prostate.[12] It is the altered hormone DHT—rather than testosterone—that actually causes prostate cells to grow. At a dose of 5 mg a day, the DHT level in the blood is reduced by 75 percent and by 80 percent in the prostate, while testosterone in the blood increases by 10 percent.[13]

The clinical goal of finasteride therapy in symptomatic BPH patients is to reduce the volume (size) of the enlarged prostate gland, increase urinary flow rate, improve the symptoms associated with bladder outlet obstruction, and halt the progression of the disease.[14] As a result of taking Proscar, then, the size of the prostate ceases to increase and may even shrink. If a man's BPH stems from muscular contractions of the enlarged prostate around the urethra, however, Proscar will have no effect.[15]

Finasteride is not effective in all patients; one reason is thought to be the presence of a 5-alpha-reductase isoenzyme in the skin that is not inhibited by finasteride, leaving incomplete hormonal blockade. Trials using inhibitors of prostate and skin isoenzymes of 5-alpha-reductase are needed to further clarify this issue.[16]

Unfortunately, for those men for whom Proscar is effective, the effect lasts only as long as the medication is being taken. If it is stopped, the prostate begins to grow again. While blocking action in the prostate, finasteride does not reduce the level of testosterone in the blood stream, allowing most men to have a normal sex drive, although decreased libido is one of the side effects for some men.[17] Other common side effects of Proscar, which may or may not disappear as the body adjusts to the medication, include a decrease in the volume of semen, and impotence.[18]

Proscar must be given for six months before its effectiveness can be assessed,[19] and for at least one year to achieve maximum prostate shrinkage. For some men the time factor is a definite disadvantage compared with the more rapid relief offered by surgery or alpha-adrenergic blockers. The efficacy of finasteride is also dependent on prostate size.[20]

A major concern of Proscar therapy for BPH is its effect on serum levels of PSA, which have been known to decrease in a range of 26 to 50 percent when a man is taking Proscar.[21] At least one study recommends that when evaluating PSA levels, doctors should double the level in finasteride-treated patients in order to allow for appropriate interpretation of PSA values and to not mask the detection of prostate cancer.[22]

One doctor recommends that before beginning finasteride treatment, a man be screened for prostatic cancer with at least a digital

A recent review of pharmacological studies suggest that Proscar is most effective in men with large prostates, while alpha-blockers such as Hytrin worked in men with both small or large prostates.

rectal exam and measurement of serum levels of PSA. If the results of either of these tests are abnormal, the man should undergo transrectal ultrasound and biopsy of the prostate before finasteride therapy is initiated.[23]

The interpretation of these studies is the subject of intense debate among urologists. Whether or not the choice of alpha-blocker therapy versus 5-alpha-reductase inhibitors should be based on prostate size is currently unclear and is unlikely to be resolved until further studies become available.[24]

Alpha-blockers seem to be more effective than finasteride during the first year of treatment, but only finasteride induces regression of the prostate and offers increased efficacy over time.[25] An analysis of the data from all available randomized trials comparing finasteride with a placebo and having a two-year follow-up, was published in 1997. The study resulted in a pooled series of 4,222 men with moderate BPH (2,113 in the finasteride group and 2,109 in the placebo group). It showed that treatment with finasteride for up to two years cuts the frequency of acute urinary retention in half (53 percent) and reduces surgical intervention by more than one-third, relative to placebo patients.[26]

A 1997 review of the published medical literature from 1994 to April 1996 indicates that finasteride produces a lower response rate and smaller improvement in voiding symptoms than surgery, and that the combination of terazosin and finasteride has not been proven to be more effective than terazosin alone. In general, alpha-adrenergic blockers (sometimes called "antagonists") exhibit a faster onset of action and produce greater improvement of voiding symptoms than does finasteride.[27]

Proscar was approved by the FDA in the summer of 1992 for treatment of BPH. In 1993, the Division of Cancer Prevention and Control of the National Cancer Institute organized the Prostate Cancer Prevention Trial (PCPT), the first-ever large-scale trial to study

A man on Proscar needs to plan on being on it for the rest of his life, which can be not only expensive (about $70+ a month, $840+ annually, as determined by a California pharmacy) but inconvenient, inasmuch as a long list of other prescription and over-the-counter drugs cannot be taken with it because of serious drug interactions. This especially includes antidepressants; antihistamines; and non-prescription medicines for appetite control, asthma, and colds (including nose drops or sprays), coughs, hay fever, or sinus problems.[28]

the prevention of prostate cancer using Proscar. It opened for participant enrollment in October 1994, with a planned three-year period to randomize the selection of 18,000 men, which it did exactly three years later, after a three-month placebo run-in period to test compliance with drug administration as well as toxicity. As the PCPT is a prevention trial, its goal was to enroll men at least 55 years old who were free of prostate cancer as determined by a normal digital rectal examination and a PSA of less than 3.0 ng/ml. Given these two factors, the statistical likelihood of a positive prostate biopsy for cancer would be less than 3 percent.[29] In fact, the actual PSA range of the men enrolled was from 0.2 to 3.0 ng/ml with a median of 1.1 ng/ml.[30]

Half of the men in the study will take one 5 mg tablet of finasteride per day for seven years; the other half will take a placebo (an inactive tablet) for the same amount of time in the double-blind study (meaning neither the men nor their doctors will know who is receiving which pill). Both a digital rectal exam and PSA will be

> *Several publications describing the Prostate Cancer Prevention Trial, which will be completed in 2004, indicate that Proscar is being used because it has an exceptionally low level of side effects and those that have been documented are comparatively mild. Although that's not the way we read its descriptions, you'll have to judge for yourself.*

performed annually. If the exam is abnormal for men in either group, or the PSA exceeds 4.0 ng/ml for men in the placebo group, a biopsy will be recommended. At the end of seven years, all participants will undergo a prostate biopsy. In addition to the primary end point of the trial, many additional side investigations will also be conducted, including a central pathology repository to house representative tissues from biopsies, and dietary and quality-of-life substudies. That 15 percent of the participants have a family history of prostate cancer will make a number of investigations possible into the genetics of the disease.[31]

CLINICAL TRIALS INVESTIGATING NEW MEDICATIONS

Many hospitals now have prostate centers that are investigating the management of BPH without surgery. If a man is willing to participate in the investigation of promising new medications not yet on the market and his condition is such that he qualifies, he may be a candidate for a hospital's ongoing clinical trial of a new drug. Medications that are researched through clinical trials are those where research has already demonstrated safety and success with laboratory animals, but where human testing is still insufficient to establish approval of the drug by the FDA.

Work on new drugs occurs constantly in research laboratories. In Japan, for instance, a new steroid inhibitor of 5-alpha-reductase, identified at present only as FR146687, is being tested on rats and beagles and appears to reduce the growth and DHT content in the prostate.[32] A second nonsteroidal 5-alpha-reductase inhibitor, FK143, is also being tested on beagles, and appears to reduce prostate volume by about the same amount as that of finasteride, and smaller than that of some other androgen receptor antagonist (nullifier) drugs being tested.[33]

Still another 5-alpha-reductase drug, GG745, is being tested in North Carolina. In laboratory studies with rats, dogs, and selective studies with men, a single dose decreased DHT levels significantly more than a single dose of finasteride, and the researchers suggest that GG745 inhibits both of the 5-alpha-reductase isoenzymes (enzymes that are chemically distinct but functionally similar) in the prostate unlike finasteride, which inhibits only one.[34]

POPULAR HERBAL SUPPLEMENTS FOR BPH

The belief that "there is no illness but that there is a plant to cure it" was "at the root of all medicine from ancient Alexandria through to Renaissance Europe," writes Sue Minter, curator of the Chelsea Physic Garden in England. "The entire countryside was nature's pharmacy."[35]

Healers wrote and illustrated medicinal handbooks known as "herbals," and planted physic gardens, which became the basis for the botanical garden of today. Columbus's return from his journeys and the successful navigation of a route to the Far East in 1498 brought new plants for cultivation to Renaissance Europe, contributing to the many herbs and plants that have a long and honored history in medicine and pharmacology. Learned men—not unlike the medicine men of primitive tribes—have long studied and used plants that would later became the focus of the numerous plant-based medications used today.[36] According to the American Medical Association, willow bark yielded salicin, the source of aspirin. Fox-glove was the source of digitalis, and snakeroot was the source of reserpine.[37]

Perhaps because of European countries long-term link to the use of herbs, phytopharmaceutical agents have been used regularly there for the treatment of BPH. When the sales of drugs for BPH treatment were recorded for various European countries, the largest sales were of finasteride, followed by plant extracts. Alpha-adrenergic blockers ranked third.[38]

In recent years there has been a prominent increase in the use of plant extracts in Germany. One of the most popular in both Germany and other European countries is an extract from the saw palmetto berry *(Serenoa repens)*. Other popular European plant remedies include the roots of the stinging nettle *(Urtica dioica),* rye pollen (one of the components of Cernitin), and pumpkin seeds.

A 1995 German report on the use of plant extracts in treating BPH, summarized in English on the Internet Medline, indicated that their effects were no better than those of placebos, especially with regard to how well they are able to block the effect of 5-alpha-reductase.[39] Two years later, however, a review of selected clinical studies, also written in German and reported summarily on Medline, indicated that pumpkin seeds (which contain zinc) and the natural extracts from several plants (especially saw palmetto and stinging nettle roots) appeared to perform better than placebos in reducing mild to moderate symptoms of BPH, but not necessarily in inhibiting further prostate growth.[40]

SAW PALMETTO (SERENOA REPENS)

Probably the best-known (and one of the most extensively researched) of the plant supplements being touted today for prostate problems is saw palmetto. Tea from the dark red berries of Serenoa, a small, scrubby palm native to the West Indies and the Atlantic coast of the United States, had long been extolled in folklore to help urinary tract infections and sexual problems such as impotency, and its use was common in the early years of the twentieth century. Although the saw palmetto was considered to have little therapeutic value by the scientific community, the *U.S. National Formulary* listed it as a drug until 1950.

Permixon, as it is known in many European countries, Saudi Arabia, and New Zealand; and Talso, as it is known in Germany, is an extract of the pulp and seeds of the dwarf palm and is a mixture of various natural compounds. Homeopathic practitioners often use a homeopathic dilution of saw palmetto called *Sabal serrulata* to treat prostatitis.

Promotion of the use of saw palmetto as an aid to BPH is based on the presumption that BPH is caused by an accumulation of testosterone in the prostate. Saw palmetto works by the same mechanism as Proscar—that is, it works by stopping the production of 5-alpha-reductase, preventing testosterone from converting to DHT. Recent laboratory studies by a group of German scientists demonstrated that it also inhibited production of 5-alpha-reductase in human BPH tissue obtained by suprapubic prostatectomy.[41] It has been suggested that saw palmetto may also inhibit DHT from binding to cellular androgen receptors[42] and thus increases its breakdown and excretion.[43]

Various studies have shown that saw palmetto is effective in reducing the urinary symptoms of BPH, even though it typically does not decrease the volume of the prostate as much as finasteride, nor change PSA levels.[44]

For instance, in one study of 110 men, saw palmetto decreased nighttime urination by 45 percent, increased urinary flow rate more than 50 percent, and reduced the amount of urine left in the bladder after urination (posturination residual volume) by 42 percent.[45] Of 305 patients taking an oral dosage of 160 mg of saw palmetto twice daily (a total of 320 mg, the typical dosage used in studies), 88 percent showed significant improvement after 90 days of treatment.[46]

In one of the largest trials conducted, more than 1,000 men were randomized to receive 160 mg of *Serenoa repens* twice daily or 5 mg of finasteride once daily for six months. No statistically significant difference was demonstrated between the two groups for patients' self-rated quality-of-life (that is, both were equally effective), while the International Prostate Symptom Score (IPPS) improved by 37 percent for those men taking *Serenoa repens* compared with 39 percent for those taking Proscar.[47]

In a second randomized, double-blind study conducted in 87 urology centers in nine European countries, of 1,098 patients originally selected, 951 patients who had BPH and symptoms of associated bladder flow obstruction completed the study. They, too, took either 160 mg of Permixon *(Seronoa repens)* morning and evening (464 men) or 5 mg Proscar each morning (484 men), as recommended by the manufacturers. To guarantee the double-blind design, patients received either Permixon plus placebo twice daily (4 tablets total) or finasteride plus placebo in the morning, with two placebos in the evening (4 tablets total).[48]

At 26 weeks, both treatments had induced similar decreases in the IPSS score (37 percent for those on Permixon; 39 percent for those on Proscar), with two-thirds of the patients responding in each treatment group. Patients receiving Proscar experienced a statistically significant deterioration in sexual function score compared to those receiving Permixon. The difference was noted in the first follow-up visit at 6 weeks and remained significant for the 26 weeks of the study. Peak urinary flow rate increased in both groups but more significantly in the finasteride group. Although both treatments reduced the size of the prostate, by 13 weeks the reduction induced by Proscar was significantly greater than that due to Permixon and remained the same at 26 weeks.[49]

One distinct advantage for the palm extract, in contrast to Proscar, is that saw palmetto has few or no significant side effects—or at least they have never been reported in clinical trials using either the extract or with direct ingestion of the berries. In contrast, Proscar users have reported side effects, the most common being gastrointestinal problems such as nausea and abdominal pain.[50] According to natural healing advocate Dr. Julian Whitaker, detailed toxicology studies on the saw palmetto extract, carried out on mice, rats, and dogs, show no toxic effects.[51]

A major problem in determining the effectiveness of saw palmetto involves the flaws in many of the studies, both pro and con, and the relatively short time during which they were carried out. In 1991, the Scientific Committee of the First International Consultation on BPH advocated that trials needed to be randomized, conducted under double-blind conditions, compared with an appropriate control (a placebo) when one drug is used, and include a follow-up of *at least one year.* The reason for the minimum of a one-year follow-up is that in most studies where placebo therapy has been used, the symptoms in both control and placebo groups have shown improvement over a short term. In addition, Proscar's efficacy is rather limited in a short-term perspective, so that when compared with Proscar in the short term, saw palmetto will usually show greater relief.[52]

Numerous saw palmetto studies can be cited where the methodology apparently lacked the requisite comprehensiveness. For example, in Italy 63 patients with BPH participated in a double-blind study to compare the efficacy of a drug known as alfuzosin with saw palmetto. The drug was found to be superior in the treatment of urinary symptoms; however, the test was of only three weeks' duration.[53] In another instance, an article in Spanish, reported on the Internet Medline, indicated that when 25 patients receiving prazosin were compared with 20 patients receiving saw palmetto for 12 weeks, prazosin was found to be slightly more effective in controlling the irritative symptoms of BPH. Unfortunately, the summary does not indicate that a placebo-control group was used, or whether the study was double-blind.[54] And, of course, these studies have the built-in problem of being short-term. They are suggestive, but not definitive.

Clearly, when the literature is reviewed, larger, randomized or double-blind trials of adequate duration are required. Furthermore, studies advocating the use of saw palmetto frequently do not present opposing evidence, which often shows conflicting results or that medications were superior. Nor do they make attempts to address the reasons for that evidence. In addition, many of the most enthusiastic recommendations for the use of saw palmetto are anecdotal (and often provided by manufacturers).

In 1990, Enzymatic Therapy, the company that introduced the saw palmetto extract into the United States, petitioned the FDA to have it approved for the treatment of BPH, but their application was rejected.[55] The FDA decided that the effects of saw palmetto did not seem meaningful enough to be an effective treatment and refused to grant over-the-counter status as a medication.[56]

PYGEUM AFRICANUM

The powdered bark of the *Pygeum* tree, a large, tropical African evergreen, has been a folk remedy for the treatment for urinary dis-

> *An extract made from the bark of the Pygeum tree, available as an over-the-counter medication in European countries and sometimes known as Tadenan, has been shown to be effective in several studies. In France, 81 percent of doctors' prescriptions for BPH are for Pygeum.*

orders for centuries. Although the *Pygeum* produces beautiful creamy white flowers and later, bright red berries, it is the tree's brown bark that the tribes of Natal have prized and long used as a cure for bladder pains and urinary difficulties.[57] Traditionally the bark was gathered, powdered, then steeped in hot water and drunk as a tea. *Pygeum* contains "phytosterols," which have anti-inflammatory properties. They work to decrease prostatic swelling, reduce harmful prostaglandins that cause prostatic inflammation, and to diminish prolactin, which, in turn, decreases the prostate's uptake of testosterone.

In one double-blind, placebo-controlled, randomized trial with 263 men in Germany, urinary symptoms improved in 66 percent of the men given the extract, compared to 31 percent of the men given a placebo. Although most side effects were minor, in two instances gastrointestinal side effects were sufficient to cause men to discontinue treatment.[58]

American urologists assert that the reports of *Pygeum*'s success are not supported by well-controlled studies. For instance, there are many short-term, nonplacebo studies that are not well constructed enough to withstand scientific scrutiny. However, an article in the July/August 1994 issue of *Natural Health* reported that when a University of Southern California professor of urology, Dr. Charles E. Shapiro, reviewed some of the European studies (we don't know which ones), he acknowledged that *Pygeum* appeared to work as effectively as Proscar or Hytrin.[59]

STINGING NETTLE (URTICA DIOICA)

In a German laboratory, various strengths of extracts of stinging nettle roots *(Urtica dioica)* were used to test the inhibition of laboratory-induced prostate growth in an adult mouse, and one of them (20 percent methanolic extract) was found to inhibit growth by 51.4 percent.[60]

At least one study has discovered that some of the steroidal components of the roots of the stinging nettle inhibit certain specific membrane and enzyme activities of the prostate, which inhibition may subsequently suppress prostate-cell metabolism and growth.[61]

Much more work needs to be done with this herb before it is ready to be considered potentially useful for treatment of BPH.

BETA-SITOSTEROLS

As we have indicated, the use of plant-derived drugs is well-established in the treatment of BPH in European countries. Nevertheless, in 1991 the International Consensus Committee on BPH declared that these drugs had not yet been studied adequately to determine their exact effectiveness and mode of action.[62] Prompted by that statement, pharmacological and clinical research on phytotherapeutic compounds for BPH intensified in an attempt to find effective, low-risk, low-cost drugs,[63] and attention was focused on the beta-sitosterols.

Beta-sitosterol products may include a mixture of agents, most of which are phytoesterols. The mechanism by which phytosterols work is still unknown. Studies testing them typically employ the ingestion of 10 to 20 mg per day, often taken three times daily. One available commercial combination is called Harzol.

Again, many of the studies have been conducted in Europe; however an American study was done in 1993 and reported in a 1995 issue of *The Lancet.* In a randomized, double-blind, placebo-controlled study, 200 patients from eight private urological practices, all with symptomatic BPH, were treated for six months with either 20 mg of beta-sitosterol (containing Harzol and a mixture of other phytosterols) three times daily, or with a placebo of the same size and shape.

After initial data were gathered, patients were assessed monthly for compliance, side effects, and modified Boyarsky scores. The International Prostate Symptom Score (IPPS) was readministered and measurements of urinary flow and prostatic volume taken at three and six months. Laboratory testing was repeated at the end of the six-month study.

Modified Boyarsky scores decreased at a statistically significant level in the beta-sitosterol-treated group compared to the placebo group. In other words, the difference could not have occurred by chance. The difference did not begin to show up until about four weeks of treatment but was consistent thereafter. IPPS decreased, quality-of-life scores improved, the peak flow rate of urine increased, and the man voiding time and the residual urinary volume decreased in those men taking the beta-sitosterol, at a statistically significant difference from their initial scores. These parameters did not change significantly for the placebo group, and the amount of difference in the changes between the two groups was also at a statistically significant level. No relevant reduction of prostatic volume occurred in either group.[64]

In Germany, a randomized, double-blind, and placebo-controlled clinical trial was conducted to assess the efficacy and safety of 130 mg (65 mg twice daily) of beta-sitosterol for the treatment of BPH. The drug used in the trial consisted of a chemically defined extract of phytosterols, known commercially as Azuprostat, and derived from several plant species (*Pinus, Picea,* or *Hyposix*), with beta-sitosterol as the main component. Between October 1993 and September 1994, a total of 177 patients were recruited at 13 private urological centers, and 155 completed the required six months of the study.

Subjective measurements included the IPPS, and a quality-of-life index, while objective measurements were peak urinary flow rate and postvoid residual urinary volume. The subjective differences between the treated and placebo groups were statistically significant. There were also significant increases in peak urinary flow rate and decreases in postvoid residual urinary volume. Nearly half of the total improvement occurred in the first month, with improvement increasing more slowly during the remaining months.[65]

It seems clear that beta-sitosterols can affect BPH symptoms just as well as some of the pharmaceutical products—and without their adverse side effects. It remains for future investigations to focus on (1) longer-term treatments with beta-sitosterol, (2) evaluation or identification of the specific compounds within the mixtures of phytosterols, and (3) on the possible biochemical mechanisms affecting symptom changes.[66]

•   •   •

Obviously, medical therapy has become increasingly important in the treatment of BPH. New surgical techniques continue to be developed and perfected. Compared with placebos, both androgen-suppressing and alpha-adrenoceptor blockade therapies are effective therapies; however, they continue to have adverse side effects for many men. Proscar must be given for six months before its effec-

> *Men who decide to discontinue any current phar-maceutical therapies because of side effects should be aware that while the side effects may disap-pear, the symptoms will also return.*

tiveness for a specific patient can be assessed, and for at least one full year to achieve maximum prostate shrinkage.

The major disadvantage of alpha-blockers is their ability to produce vasodilation leading to dizziness, postural hypotension, and fainting or loss of consciousness. In addition they commonly produce sleepiness, heart palpitations, and nasal congestion.[67]

Although these are the usual nonsurgical options that most urologists will recommend to a patient with BPH, there is another option. Now it's time, in the next chapter, to compare the research and effects of the Prostate Cure to the other treatments for BPH that we've examined. We think you'll be impressed with the results, but we'll let the research speak for itself.

4

THE MIRACLE OF CERNITIN

What is Cernitin?

*

Who discovered the link between flower pollen and BPH?

*

How does Cernitin work?

*

How much Cernitin is recommended?

*

How and where has Cernitin been researched and tested?

*

Why is Cernitin so little-known in America?

The development of Cernitin is a story of remarkable fortitude and determination. It is a fascinating look into how scientific discoveries can be developed through the hard work
and determination of men and women—and with a little luck. It is
the story of how two remarkable men were determined to overcome
all obstacles in creating a new treatment for men with BPH.

The Cernitin story begins in the beautiful Swedish village of
Grevie in the spring of 1950. Åke Asplund had been a railroad
man since 1934 and was working as the stationmaster in Grevie.[1]
Although Grevie was a small community, it was a center for the collection and distribution of eggs; hence, the need for a railway stop.

It was at this time that Åke met Gösta Carlsson, another railway worker. Gösta's hobby was beekeeping, which he had learned from his father. Gösta had the unusual idea of collecting pollen directly from flowers in order to feed it to his bees early in the spring—a meal that set off a flurry of activity and growth in his hive populations. Early feeding meant that the queen bee started her production of eggs earlier, resulting in a new generation of bees ready to collect pollen sooner, and an increased production of honey in the colony. Who wouldn't want that?

The enthusiasm of the two men led them to write a book— *Rationell Biskötsel* (Rational Beekeeping)—as a promotional effort to encourage other Swedish beekeepers to buy pollen from them for their own bees. To their dismay, Åke and Gösta found that Swedish beekeepers were not the least bit interested in their ideas. They did not give up, however, and used their disappointment to promote a new product.

Since his youth, Åke had been an active participant in a group interested in a healthy lifestyle. The group camped out in the summer, cycled and walked long distances together, and trained in a homemade gymnasium. Åke was the district secretary of the local association and knew many people in the health movement, who expressed an interest in eating natural products as food or food supplements. Some had started their own shops to sell various kinds of "health foods," or sold natural products as food or food supplements, and were interested in promoting new products.

So Åke and Gösta began making a mixture of 70 percent honey and 30 percent pure flower pollen, which they packed in glass jars and called Pollisan. They marketed the product to health-minded friends and health food stores, largely through a company called A. B. Anjo, formed by two friends of Åke's.

FIRE: THE FIRST SETBACK

Housed in a four-story wooden barn, the business grew slowly but steadily for about five years. Then, on September 15, 1952, disaster struck. Arriving at the plant that morning on his motorbike, Gösta discovered that a fire had broken out sometime during the night and had not only destroyed the building, but all of their original equipment—including some built to Gösta's unique and secret designs. Gösta initially panicked because he realized he had not paid the fire insurance premium; however, Åke had used money from his wife's dowry to pay it.

Still the most devastating blow came when the two men realized that the fire had also consumed their entire stock of pollen. You may ask yourself, as did the police who investigated the scene, what's the loss of a little pollen? But the loss was anything but "little." The two men had managed to acquire 600 kilograms of pollen, valued at 6.5 million Swedish crowns (at the time, one U.S. dollar equaled about 5.5 Swedish crowns).

FROM THE ASHES . . . A NEW BUSINESS

Eventually Åke and Gösta received a payment from their insurance company, and some financial help from friends. Count von Geijer of Vegeholm, the owner of the estate on which the barn had been located, agreed to finance the design and construction of a new building to meet Åke and Gösta's exact requirements. They were back in business.

By July 4, 1953, they were ready to open their new facility. Although the two men had sold their Pollisan through A. B. Anjo, with the completion of the new construction they decided to form their own company. They named it Cernelle. And, as Åke writes in his autobiography, now that they had the opportunity to develop totally new products from flower pollen, they also had many questions: Was it possible to develop a product or products from flower pollen that might be useful as medicine? What secrets were still hidden in the small pollen grains? Obviously much research was necessary. A more practical and pressing question facing the two men was: How do we market new, unknown, and as yet undeveloped products?[2]

For some time a pharmaceutical laboratory in Stockholm, A. B. Kabi, well-known in Sweden as one of the most advanced manufacturers of penicillin, had been in contact with the men. Officers at A. B. Kabi were considering the idea of not only conducting research on pollen chemistry but also working on the problem of how to transform pollen into dragées, small tablet-like balls. Now A. B. Kabi began manufacturing dragées for Cernelle, which it marketed under the name Cernelle Pollendragées. Unlike bee pollen, which bees have treated with their saliva and in which other pollutants can be present, the pure flower pollen from Cernelle was free from toxic substances.

In 1955, the small private company owned by the two men became a subsidiary company of A. B. Kabi and was renamed A. B. Cernelle. Still, it remained largely a family affair, as wives, nieces and nephews, and the wives and children of neighbors gathered pollen directly from flowers, eventually harvesting several tons for the new company.

Åke and Gösta began to test the effects of feeding their product to bees and other animals, and learned that they grew faster and that bees, especially, grew larger. The company began to develop new health-food-oriented products. Now that the two men had the expertise and knowledge to collect pollen on a large scale and knew how to purify and treat it for storage, they decided they wanted to produce their own tablets rather than continue to buy them from A. B. Kabi.

In 1958 they hired an experienced Estonian pharmacist living in Sweden, Dr. E. P. Tonisson, to set up a production plant in Vegeholm. They converted an abandoned farmhouse into a factory and began to manufacture Pollitabs, a new product to replace Pollendragées.

All the while, they continued their research on the effects of feeding pollen to animals. Bees grew larger with the addition of extra pollen to their diet. Chickens and rats increased in weight faster, and fewer died when the pollen was added to their diet. Marketing visits to health food stores indicated shopkeepers and customers wanted a wider range of products, and the company began developing additional products.

POLLEN POWER

About this time Åke met a talented scientist, Dr. Hans Palmstierna, who was working at the famous Karolinska Institute in Stockholm. Dr. Palmstierna, a doctor of medicine and also a microbiologist, was interested in reducing the allergenic qualities of pollen and pollen extracts.

Here was a trained expert who not only understood Åke's and Gösta's dream regarding the expanded possibilities of flower pollen, but who also brought solid knowledge and scientific expertise to the subject. In short order, he showed the men that though pollen grains are minuscule, they are nevertheless covered by an almost insoluble sheath that cannot be assimilated by humans. The tiny husk itself is covered by a thin layer of mucus where bacteria and fungi can thrive, and which some believe may be the major source of many pesky springtime allergies. So the next step was to find a way to either remove the sheath or to extract the pollen from inside the sheath.

Dr. Palmstierna spent his summers and holidays at the plant developing methods of extracting the active ingredient from the pollen—much as bees do when they make royal jelly for their queen. Dr. Palmstierna used water and oil solvents: one extract contained water-soluble components, one contained fat-soluble components.

The fat-soluble component was found to be nonallergic, while the other contained allergenic substances. In addition, the men learned how to spray-dry the extracts to make them stable and suitable for use in tablets.

In one of those coincidental occurrences that have long-ranging consequences, a well-known Swedish physician, Professor Erik Ask-Upmark, who suffered regularly from prostatitis, had began using the tablets at the urging of his wife after she revived a sick pigeon by feeding it crushed pollen tablets in water. Mrs. Ask-Upmark was convinced the product would help her husband, too.

Dr. Ask-Upmark began to experiment on himself, varying the dosages and strengths of the extract. At his request, the company made a stronger tablet just for him, called—you guessed it—Cernitin. Remarkably, the doctor's symptoms disappeared. Being a scientist and somewhat skeptical, Dr. Ask-Upmark wondered if the change was really caused by the Cernitin. A serendipitous bit of forgetfulness soon convinced him that it was.

On a trip to England to deliver a presentation, the doctor failed to bring his Cernitin. Within days the inflammation returned, and, leaving the conference early, he hurried back to Sweden and his Cernitin tablets. Four days later his symptoms were gone, and the now-convinced doctor began to prescribe Cernitin to his patients afflicted with prostatitis. In 1960, Professor Ask-Upmark published the first paper supporting the use of Cernitin in a Swedish medical journal.[3]

THE WORD SPREADS

When the doctor published his findings that the pollen extract worked to eliminate prostatic symptoms, many doctors were doubtful, because this was the report of only a single case. But a few urologists were interested, and their early results also were highly encouraging.

A professor from the University of Lund, Gösta Jönsson, tried Cernitin on 10 patients with prostatitis, among them three who had been treated with other forms of therapy for five years with no improvement. After treatment with Cernitin, all were symptom-free. Again, the medical community expressed doubts, and rightly so, because Professor Jönsson had no control group with which to compare his patients.[4]

In 1962 a second urologist, Dr. Gösta Leander, instituted the first double-blind study of Cernitin, using 61 patients with prostatitis. Members of one group received the Cernitin, while the others received a placebo tablet having a similar taste. Both groups continued to receive the so-called conservative treatment that was standard at the time—massaging the prostate to eliminate adhesions and stimulate blood flow. "Conservative," maybe, but it was a thoroughly unpleasant procedure. As one urologist reported, patients were often "disinclined to complete the treatment." Thus, it was with considerable pleasure that Dr. Leander was able to report that those who received the combined conservative treatment plus Cernitin had an increased normalization rate of almost 50 percent compared to those with conservative treatment alone. Dr. Leander observed virtually no side effects.[5]

As more and more doctors began to use Cernitin, the company grew, and by 1960 it had 15 employees. Now it became apparent that A. B. Cernelle—which was not registered as a pharmaceutical company in Sweden—needed to be. Early in 1961 the company applied for registration.

Keep in mind that 12 years had now passed since Åke and Gösta met and began the development and promotion of pure flower pollen. A. B. Cernelle continued to grow, building a new factory near the town of Engelholm to manufacture its tablets, and installing a cold-storage room to house its stock of pollen. The company also built a hall for processing the collected pollen.

In 1963, Cernelle organized a symposium on urology in Helsingborg, inviting doctors from Sweden, Denmark, Switzerland, and Germany. German scientists and urologists began to enthusiastically use Cernitin for prostatitis, as did physicians in other countries. Soon there were more than 80 reports of clinical, pharmacological, and chemical studies, all but one showing some improvement—mostly subjective—and none showing any side effects (as contrasted to antibiotic treatments, which ran the risk, as they still do, of producing intestinal disorders, allergic reactions, and resistant bacteria).

Many battles with banks, government regulators, and bureaucrats—not to mention the threat of bankruptcy—beset the company over the next decades. But restructuring, foreign growth, and vision kept Cernelle afloat. In the early 1970s, Gösta Carlsson formed another company, Allergon, which he subsequently sold to Pharmacia. Because of this split, there are now two companies that produce the raw material used in flower pollen extract, Cernelle and Allergon. These products used in treating BPH in men are marketed in the United States under the names Cernitin by Cernelle and Prostaphil by Allergon, and will be widely available in drug and health food stores.

Copious amounts of research have now been conducted on Cernitin, and we are therefore very confident of its effectiveness. The manufacturers at Allergon assure us that their product, Prostaphil, is essentially similar to Cernitin. However, because we have not seen any research comparing the two products, we cannot assure readers that the two are indeed identical.

Brenda Adderly, the coauthor of this book, comes across this dilemma frequently when asked about the efficacy and quality of one product over another. Usually this arises in a product category where quality varies widely and there is no way the consumer can tell the poor products from the good ones.

As a result, in the near future Brenda will be having products analyzed for quality by a respected independent laboratory affiliated with a major university. Then (much as *Good Housekeeping* does), she'll permit companies whose products are deemed to be of superior quality to put her "seal of approval" onto their packaging. Obviously, she is not saying that if her seal doesn't appear the product is necessarily inferior. However, if it *does* appear, you can be certain that product is everything it claims to be.

Brenda will also keep readers informed about any new research on flower pollen extract and treating enlarged prostates in her newsletter, *Health Watch,* and on the Web at www.BrendaAdderly.com.

DRUG STATUS, DOSAGE AND WORLDWIDE ACCEPTANCE

Today, Cernelle's flower pollen extract is distributed throughout Europe and in Malaysia, Singapore, Hong Kong, Thailand, Japan, and Taiwan. The Japanese distributor also supports much clinical research work and pharmacological tests on Cernitin for the treatment of prostatic disorders. Åke Asplund reports that several studies conducted in Japan showed that Cernitin inhibited the increase in prostate weight in BPH, and that the two active components in Cernitin (fat- and water-soluble) act respectively to stimulate the muscles of the bladder and to "act on the urinary tube and outlet and thus support the flow of urine."[6]

Even though Cernitin is a 100 percent natural product, like any drug it has been carefully scrutinized for safety and toxicity issues.

Cernitin has achieved drug status in six countries (Switzerland, Germany, Austria, Japan, South Korea, and Argentina). Two of these, Germany and Switzerland, have rigorous approval processes and are therefore looked upon favorably by the U.S. Food and Drug Administration.

Significantly, there is no lethal dose of Cernitin. Toxicity studies have shown it to be incredibly safe—animal tests at one thousand times the strength of human dosage showed no adverse effects. Nine separate international studies were conducted, and nearly 3,000 men took Cernitin for periods ranging from four weeks to six months. Again, Cernitin proved safe and effective. It is druglike in its efficacy, yet is a natural compound bereft of side effects.

Although all of the specific actions of Cernitin are not known, scientists have been able to determine the three main beneficial components of Cernitin's activity. The first is Cernitin's anti-inflammatory properties, which act to reduce engorgement of the tissues of the prostate by blocking the formation of inflammatory chemicals. Second, Cernitin exhibits smooth-muscle relaxation properties in the bladder and prostate region; this means that urine flow through the urethra is improved. Finally, Cernitin affects the metabolism of DHT, the male hormone that is a significant factor in the development of BPH. Specifically, it inhibits the production of DHT, which, in turn, inhibits prostate growth.

Most of the research that has been done on Cernitin comes from the many studies conducted in European countries. It is from some of these that we learn more specifically the contents of a tablet of Cernitin.[7] Most research relies on a standard dosage form of 63 mg of Cernitin per tablet, with the standard dosage of two to three tablets twice a day.

The water-soluble Cernitin T 60 and the oily (acetone-soluble) Cernitin GBX are in a ratio of 20 to 1 in a standard dosage (e.g., 60 mg T60 to 3 mg GBX).[8] Cernitin GBX and Cernitin T-60 are extracts of a mixture of eight different pollen strains from plant species grown in southern Sweden, namely timothy, maize, rye, hazel, sallow, aspen, oxeye daisy, and pine.[9] Previous research showed that Cernitin GBX consists of three beta-sitosterols.[10]

CERNITIN PROVES ITS EFFECTIVENESS

As we've stated, a plethora of studies from foreign countries have investigated the efficacy of flower pollen extract in the treatment and eradication of the symptoms of BPH. Here we will summarize some of the most impressive and relevant studies.

One of the oldest is a fully controlled study that was conducted in 1967 by Professors Masaaki Ohkoshi, Nabuo Kawamura, and Ichiron Nagakubo of Keio University in Japan.[11] In this study, Cernitin was administered to 14 patients with prostatitis or nongonorrheal urethritis, and placebos to 16 patients. In 10 Cernitin cases, the treatment was successful; in three others, slightly effective; and in one case, ineffective. In the placebo group, seven found treatment to be effective and nine observed no change. No side effects were experienced in either the test or the control group.

In an inhouse, privately published study conducted for Tobishi Pharmaceutical Co., Ltd. (the Japanese distributor of Cernitin) by medical doctors from the Department of Urology at the Kyoto University School of Medicine, 24 patients with BPH were seen at the school's outpatient clinic.[12] Cernitin was administered in doses of four tablets once daily in the morning, during periods ranging from 25 to 150 days. Other drugs were not employed. Complete followup was available in only 12 cases, and this only in regard to subjective symptoms and urinary retention before, during, and at the completion of the study.

Results were evaluated as "effective" for five cases (41.7 percent), "slightly effective" for five cases, and "ineffective" for two cases (16.7 percent). Two of the five "effective" cases subsequently underwent prostatectomies because their symptoms returned after withdrawal of Cernitin. One of the "slightly effective" cases also had a prostatectomy. Side effects were not experienced by any of the men.

In the discussion of their research, the doctors in this early study described some of the problems researchers experience in evaluating the success of new drugs or medications on BPH. These include (among others) the unexplained disappearance or remission of symptoms without specific treatment, and the fact that clinical symptoms do not always correlate to prostatic size—all of which make it difficult to decide what criteria should be used for evaluation. They conclude, as do other researchers, that "drugs" are usable for treatment of BPH if they can improve subjective symptoms without side effects and can be employed for long-term administration.

As another preliminary step in evaluating the effectiveness of Cernitin for Japanese men with BPH, a small study involving 25 men, chosen at random from the Tokyo Medical and Dental Hospital, was reported in 1981. The men received two tablets each of Cernitin three times a day for three months. The ages of the men in the study ranged from 53 to 77 years, with an average age of 67. Both the subjective opinions of the men and objective symptoms were evaluated. The chief complaints of the men were difficulty in urinating, frequency, and residual urine sensation.

The overall effectiveness for the mens' subjective symptoms was 64 percent, with 8 percent showing marked effectiveness, 56 percent effective, 20 percent no change, and 16 percent experiencing a deterioration of symptoms.

The table on the opposite page shows the actual percentage of improvement for each of the subjective symptoms.

The overall effectiveness of the treatment for the objective symptoms (actual residual urine, size of prostate gland, maximum urine

Symptom	Percentage of Improvement with Cernitin
Prolonged micturition difficulty	54%
Nocturnal frequency	50%
Feeling of residual urine	50%
Decrease in force of urine stream	47%
Straining during urination	41%
Delayed micturition	22%

flow rate, urethral pressure) was: effective, 36 percent; no change, 42 percent: and ineffective, 12 percent. None of the 25 patients complained of adverse effects from the use of Cernitin.

During the late 1980s and early 1990s, research on the use of Cernitin for BPH began in earnest in Japan. A multiple-center, double-blind study was performed to compare the effectiveness of Cernitin to a drug called Paraprost. Several groups of patients, totaling 192 in all, were studied for various changes and rate of effectiveness. Of the 192 patients, 159 were evaluated for the overall effect, 178 were rated on the overall safety of the drugs, and the rate of effectiveness was measured for 159 patients. They were evaluated by committee judgment, by physicians' judgment, and by changes in objective symptoms at the completion of the four-week study.

Cernitin made a higher difference in residual urinary volume, average flow rate, maximum flow rate, and prostatic weight than Paraprost. Both committee members and physicians judged the effectiveness of Cernitin to be in the 40 to 49 percent range (41.2 percent by the committee, 49.4 percent by the physicians), compared to 41.2 percent by the committee and 46.3 percent by the physicians for the Paraprost group. Although the results suggested that Cernitin was an effective drug for BPH, the differences between the two groups were not statistically significant. No side effects or abnormalities were found in the Cernitin group.[13]

Cernitin has also been researched and used in Germany for the treatment of both chronic prostatitis and BPH. In 1986 a prominent German medical doctor/researcher initiated a mammoth effort to evaluate the progress of 1,189 patients taking Cernitin.[14] Based on the diagnoses given by their 170 urologists, the men were divided into three groups: 583 men (25.4 percent) with chronic prostatitis, 590 men (25.8 percent) with BPH accompanied by prostatitis, and 1,116 men (48.4 percent) with BPH alone. The pollen-extract treatment was provided in 84 percent of the cases with a dosage of three tablets twice a day in the first week, and continued in 78.5 percent of the men with the same dosage for up to 12 weeks. Palpation, and measures of residual urine volume, peak urine flow, urine volume voided, flow time, and leukocytes (white blood cells, the presence of which indicates infection) in prostatic secretions were taken at the beginning and end of treatment.

Improvement or eradication of symptoms occurred in 64 to 82 percent of the men, depending on their respective complaints. A significant reduction in prostate size was found in 55.9 percent of those patients from the chronic prostatitis group who had an initially enlarged prostate.

Peak urine flow rate increased significantly in all three groups. Concomitantly the amount of urine voided increased, and the flow time was reduced. Side effects of slight and temporary gastrointestinal disturbances were described in 66 cases (2.9 percent), and in 1.2 percent of the cases treatment was stopped.[15]

The general assessment of the pollen-extract therapy was "good" to "very good" by 72.2 percent of the physicians and by 75 percent of the patients.

In 1986, H. Bräuer of the German research firm "Medical Service," recognizing that with an aging population BPH was becoming ever more significant, decided to study whether Cernitin or beta sitosterol was the more effective treatment for BPH. Thirty-nine patients with BPH, living in what the researchers called an "old people's home," participated in a study to compare the efficacy of the two products in treating their disorder. In the double-blind, parallel study the 19 randomized members of Group A received Cernitin, while 20 participants randomized to Group B received 10 mg of beta-sitosterol. None of the members of the groups took any additional medication. All the participants required treatment and had been receiving medical therapy for their prostatic symptomatology for more than six months with unsatisfactory results. In order to exclude possible uncheckable drug effects, a one-week, wash-out period was included before the start of the study for four men.

Both groups took two tablets three times daily for the first week, then one tablet three times a day for days 8 to 42. This study was especially important because it measured two reliable markers of BPH, namely the levels of prostatic acid phosphatase (PAP) and prostate-specific antigen (PSA). PAP is a highly tissue-specific enzyme that is normally passed from the prostate to the seminal fluid. All pathological changes of the prostate, whether cancer, BPH, or prostatitis lead to an increase in the concentration of this enzyme in the blood. PSA (more about this antigen in Chapter 8) originates from the excretory ducts of the glandular complex of the prostate and is normally present in the blood in very low concentrations but increases markedly in the presence of cellular lesions of the excretory ducts resulting from BPH. Blood, PAP, and PSA samples were taken at the beginning and the completion of the study. Other data evaluated included clinical symptoms and complaints, residual urine amounts, and bacterial cultures obtained from urine samples.

In general, comparison of the initial findings with those at the end of the study showed improvements in the clinical symptoms for both preparations, which were clearly more pronounced with the

Cernitin, according to the investigating physician's impression and those of the patients themselves.

At the beginning of the study, the residual urine volume was 35 ml for Group B and 28 ml for Group A. In both groups, the mean values had fallen to under 15 ml at the end of treatment. The parameters indicating disturbances of renal function (namely creatinine and blood urea nitrogen), also showed a clear decrease under both Cernitin and beta-sitosterol.

More important, the fall in the values of those enzyme values that indicated cellular lesions was significant, and was more pronounced in the Cernitin group. This conclusion is drawn from the reduction in PAP and PSA values. In Group A, the PAP concentration dropped significantly from 3.5 to 2.7 ng/ml, while Group B had an initial fall form 4.4 to 3.7 ng/ml, but remained at this level throughout the study. PSA concentration was lowered only 0.5 ng/ml for Group B (from 12.9 to 12.4), while it fell 2.45 ng/ml for Group A (from 8.25 to 5.8), a statistically significant decrease.

As a result, Dr. Bräuer, a meticulous German researcher prone to understatement, permitted himself to venture "that the cellular lesions of the glandular tissue resulting from the prostatic changes show marked improvement under treatment with pollen extract.[11] Considering its source, this was high praise indeed. In a rare show of true enthusiasm, the doctor added, "We consider very important the fact that the preparation is extremely well-tolerated."[16] In 1988, the efficacy and tolerability of Cernitin for treatment of BPH was investigated by Professor H. Becker, head of the Department of Urology at the Marienhospital in Hamburg, and Dr. L. Ebeling of the pharmaceutical firm Pharma Stroschein. A double-blind, placebo-controlled study was carried out over 12 weeks in six urological practices on a total of 96 patients ranging in age from 42 to 85 years. The men were split between test and control groups. The median duration of BPH had been 10 months, and BPH had been treated previously in 40.6 percent of the cases. Patients previously treated entered a four-week wash-out phase before taking either the placebo or Cernitin. The dosage for both groups was three capsules three times daily.

For those taking Cernitin, nocturia–the need to urinate during the night and the leading symptom reported by 96.9 percent of the men–significantly improved in 68.8 percent of the cases, compared with 37.2 percent using the placebo medication.

Absence of the symptoms of daytime frequency and sense of residual urine volume of those taking Cernitin also increased significantly, as shown in the following chart:

Freedom from Symptom	*Cernitin-N*	*Placebo*
Daytime frequency	48.8%	19.5%
Feeling of residual urine	37.1%	7.7%

The use of Cernitin led to a significant and continuous reduction of residual urine volume, whereas in the placebo group the residual urine after 12 weeks had increased from the 6-week value. Although prostate enlargement, as detected by palpation, decreased for 17.4 percent of the men in the Cernitin group, 10.6 percent of the patients in the placebo group also showed a decrease, a difference that could not be considered statistically significant. The same was true for prostate congestion, also measured by palpation. Congestion for men in the Cernitin group decreased by 88.5 percent; however, the congestion of men in the placebo group also decreased by 69 percent. Only one person using Cernitin reported nausea as a side effect.[17] It is not unusual in research for a certain number or percentage of persons taking a placebo to show the same results as those taking the experimental medication or procedure. The trick in research is to have that difference between the experimental and the control group show up as so substantially large as to not be attributable to chance (i.e., statistically significant).

Following the double-blind phase of the study, 92 of the patients involved in the first study from both groups were treated with Cernitin in an open trial design for 12 weeks; that is, the placebo group now received Cernitin and the treatment group from the first study continued to receive Cernitin.

In the group of 45 patients who made the change-over from the placebo to Cernitin therapy, there was a marked decrease of symptoms. For instance, after the first 12 weeks nocturia improved for only 37.2 percent of this group, whereas after the second 12 weeks—when they began taking Cernitin—the symptom improved for 68.2 percent of the men.

For other symptoms, there were similar jumps in improvement, as shown in the following table:

Symptom	Percentage of Improvement When Taking Placebo	Percentage of Improvement After Began Taking Cernitin
Dysuria (painful urination)	37.0%	60.9%
Feeling of residual urine	46.2%	65.4%
Daytime urge to urinate	62.2%	84.2%
Malaise	44.4%	74.1%

In the patients treated first with Cernitin and continuing for the next 12 weeks, the findings were slight when compared with the corresponding results in the placebo-Cernitin group, but there were no reversals in results. Side effects of pressure over the stomach and nausea occurred for three patients.[18]

At the University Hospital of Wales in Cardiff, doctors and researchers were looking for alternative treatments with fewer side effects than those associated with the known pharmacological agents used for BPH. Sixty patients, ranging in age from 56 to 89 years, with outflow obstruction due to BPH, began the double-blind, placebo-controlled study (three were excluded after initial assessment). Because of emergencies requiring surgery, 53 patients remained (29 in the Cernitin group and 24 in the placebo group) who could be evaluated at the end of six months.

Men in the Cernitin group took two capsules daily, probably a triple-strength capsule of 189 mg for six months, and the others received a nonactive compound. Evaluations were made before the study, at three months, and again at the conclusion of the study. Patients were evaluated for urine flow rate, voided volume, ultrasound measurement of residual urine, and ultrasound measurement of prostate size.

Subjective ratings based on a modified Boyarsky scoring scale for the symptoms of frequency, hesitancy, urgency, intermittency, incomplete emptying, terminal dribbling, and dysuria (painful urination), showed a statistically significant overall improvement with Cernitin (69 percent of the patients) compared to the placebo group (29 percent). On Cernitin, 57 percent of patients showed significant improvement in bladder emptying, compared with only 10 percent in the placebo group, a statistically significant difference. Concurrently, residual urine volume decreased significantly in those men receiving Cernitin, compared with the placebo group, for whom it increased.

Nocturia also improved at a statistically significant level, with 60 percent of the patients on Cernitin improved or symptom-free, compared with 30 percent of the patients on the placebo. Ultrasound showed a significant decrease in the anterior-posterior diameter of the prostate for the Cernitin group; however, differences of peak urine flow rate and voided volume were not significant (perhaps due to low subject numbers).

The percentage of other improvements experienced by the men, which were not statistically significant (meaning the differences could have occurred by chance), but which did show differences between the men taking Cernitin and those taking a placebo, are shown in the following chart:

Symptoms	Cernitin	Placebo
Daytime frequency	37%	47%
Hesitancy	47%	29%
Urgency	71%	45%
Intermittency	52%	33%
Terminal dribble	61%	56%
Dysuria (Painful discharge of urine)	62%	71%

No adverse side effects were reported, and there were no significant changes in serum cholesterol, triglycerides, or lipoproteins (molecules that transport fats throughout the body). The doctors concluded that Cernitin has a place in the treatment of patients with mild or moderate symptoms of outflow obstruction.[19]

In 1993 a team of researchers completed a controlled study of the effects of Cernitin on 90 German men with BPH, nonbacterial prostatitis, and prostatodynia. The men were divided into two groups: those without associated complicating factors, and those with complicating factors (e.g., urethral strictures, prostatic calculi, bladder neck sclerosis). Both groups took one tablet three times a day for six months and were evaluated after three and six months of treatment. In the group without complicating factors, 56 men (78 percent) had a favorable response. Twenty-six (36 percent) of the men were relieved of their symptoms. Thirty (42 percent) showed an improvement in their urine flow rate, a decrease in white blood cells in post-prostate massage urine, and a decrease in certain components in their semen. Because only one patient in the group of men with complicating factors responded to Cernitin treatment, the researchers suggest that doctors of patients who do not respond to Cernitin look for complicating factors before deciding that Cernitin is ineffective.[20]

Researchers at Leighton Hospital in Crewe, England, tried Cernitin with 15 patients who were diagnosed as having chronic prostatitis or prostatodynia. Only two patients failed to respond, while the 13 others experienced either complete relief of symptoms or a marked improvement.[21]

In 1995 researchers at the Osaka Municipal Juso Citizens' Hospital in Japan used Cernitin extract to treat 79 patients who had BPH. Patient ages ranged from 62 to 89 years. Cernitin was administered three times daily for more than four months. Subjective symptom scores decreased, as did the residual urine volume. Urine maximum flow rate and average flow rates increased. Although there was no change in prostatic volume for this group, 28 patients treated for more than one year showed a substantial decrease. No adverse reactions were observed. In the larger group, poor or insignificant results occurred in 15 percent of the patients. The doctors concluded that the overall clinical efficacy was 85 percent.[22]

In 1996, a researcher at the Central Clinical Hospital in Warsaw, Poland, divided a group of 89 patients with BPH into a group of 51 who received Cernitin and 38 who received a drug called Tadenan. Subjective improvement was reported by 78 percent of the patients in the Cernitin group, compared to 55 percent in the Tadenan-treated group. The Cernitin-treated patients experienced improvement in the urine flow rate. Decreases in residual urine and in prostate volume were also found.[23]

CANCER RESEARCH USING CERNITIN

Early in 1990 a team of researchers at Western General Hospital in Edinburgh, Scotland, used nine human-derived cancer and non-cancer cell lines to evaluate the relative in vitro (outside the living body, in an artificial environment) activity of Cernitin T-60 on cancer tissue. Of the nine cancer cell samples, only the growth of those derived from the human prostate were inhibited by Cernitin. Non-prostate-derived cancer cells showed only variable degrees of resistance. Stromal cells showed greater sensitivity than epithelial prostate cells derived from the same BPH tissue.[24]

Some of the members of this team, along with researchers in the Department of Medical Biochemistry at the University of Geneva in Switzerland, continued this work, attempting to identify an active component in Cernitin that was primarily responsible for inhibiting the growth of prostate cancer cells. They found a water-soluble ingredient that they named "FV-7," which constitutes only about one percent of the total T-60 extract.

High resolution mass spectrometry identified FV-7 as hydroxamic acid, an acid-based inhibitor. Using the initials of its components, the researchers came up with the name DIBOA to identify a synthetic extract of FV-7. Then they synthesized a sample of DIBOA in the laboratory. After determining that the composition of the synthetic DIBOA was indistinguishable from the natural FV-7, they compared the effects of the two on the growth of prostate cancer cells grown in the laboratory. Both the natural and the synthetic product slowed down cancer growth even after one day of exposure.

They were almost identical in their effect, although the inhibitory activity of the natural product, FV-7, was slightly more potent.[25]

Their research was continued, once more, at the Western General Hospital in Edinburgh, Scotland, where again the investigations of some of the members of the same team, plus others, were able to demonstrate that FV-7 inhibited the growth of DU145 prostate cancer cells and also inhibited the growth of stroma and epithelial prostate cells, although the latter required higher concentrations of FV-7 than what was required to inhibit the growth of DU145 cells.[26]

Unfortunately, no additional studies on the effect of Cernitin on cancer have been conducted, but those that were completed show that at least one component of Cernitin, FV-7, has the capacity to inhibit the growth of prostate cancer cells when applied directly to tissue in the laboratory. These studies hint that treatment involving direct application in the human body, or concentrated products of FV-7 taken orally, may eventually be possible. More research will obviously be needed to reach a definitive conclusion.

WHAT THESE STUDIES TELL US

Taken all together, studies conducted by Åke Asplund and his staff, and by independent medical researchers around the world, show Cernitin, a standardized pollen extract, to be exceptionally effective in the treatment of BPH. Unlike most drugs used to treat this condition, Cernitin is a natural product with few or no side effects or allergic reactions, and it demonstrates an effectiveness equal to or often exceeding the results achieved by prescribed medications. In fact, Cernitin frequently succeeds in situations where other drugs or treatments have failed, and it may be the treatment of choice in intractable cases of prostatitis.

Using Cernitin reduces most of the major subjective symptoms of BPH (e.g., urinary urgency and frequency) as well as objectively measurable symptoms, such as reduction in the size of the prostate, an increase in the amount of bladder emptying, and increase in peak urine flow rate. Further, it contains potent phytonutrients that help to strengthen and support the body's immune system and possibly slow down or inhibit the growth of cancer cells.

WHY CERNITIN IS SO LITTLE-KNOWN IN AMERICA

It's rather astonishing, but the fact is that while Cernitin has been widely researched abroad—and is now used in nearly every country except the United States—it is virtually unknown here. At least until now, with the publication of *The Prostate Cure.*

There are a number of reasons for this, but fortunately, the situation is changing. Let's look at how this scenario developed and what's happening with Cernitin in the United States today.

SUSPICION OF ALTERNATIVE TECHNIQUES
BY MEDICAL COMMUNITY

For years a negative attitude has prevailed among the traditional medical community in the United States toward all forms of alternative medicine, even though for years physicians themselves have been indicating the need for a broader understanding of illness.[27] Recently, however, the high cost of medical treatment (especially surgery), coupled with an enlightened consumer base interested in and using alternative medicines—often as a less invasive choice or one with fewer side effects—have begun to steadily exert their influence on traditional care, and on the medical profession itself. Acceptance has nevertheless been painfully slow. For instance, in 1988 the American Medical Association published a book entitled *Alternative Therapies, Unproven Methods & Health Fraud.* It covered 18 topics in 47 pages. By 1993 the AMA had changed the name of the publication to *Reader's Guide to Alternative Health Methods.* It included eight times as much information as before, and though there was "pro" and "con" information about many of the topics, the book still had the weighty and skeptical subtitle, "An analysis of more than 1,000 reports on unproven, disproved, controversial, fraudulent, quack and/or otherwise questionable approaches to solving health problems."[28] Among the topics included are acupuncture, ayurvedic medicine, chiropractic herbs, holistic medicine, and many, many others.

At present any treatment that is not the conventional type of treatment we expect to receive in a doctor's office (e.g., shots, medications, surgery) is typically lumped under the catchall term "alternative medicine," a term for which no adequate definition exists. Part of the difficulty is that the various systems that fall under this catchall phrase often have quite diverse philosophical, social, and cultural backgrounds.

The use of herbs and natural substances for healing is placed in the alternative medicine category in the United States, although many of them have been used and well accepted in other cultures as a standard or "traditional" form of folk medicine. Even the AMA admits that folk medicine is not generally considered to be quackery so long as it is not done for gain.[29] It includes in the category of folk medicine self-treatment, family home treatment, neighborly medical advice, and the noncommercial activities of folk healers.

According to the World Health Organization, between 65 and 80 percent of the world's population (about 3 billion people) rely on some form of culturally traditional medicine as their primary form of health care.[30] Frequently, when a healing or herbal substance from folk medicine comes to the United States, it is then classified as "alternative."

Most alternative medicine techniques combine a deep belief in the healing power of nature and the body's natural ability to heal, with a belief in "holistic" treatment; that is, focusing on the whole person (body, mind, and spirit) and on the effect of the mind-body interaction in both the production of symptoms and their cure.

According to Dr. J. Warren Salmon, professor and coordinator of the Health Specialization program in the School of Urban Policy and Planning at the University of Chicago, this broader "metaphysical" understanding of the concept of "energy" (called "chi" by the Chinese and "prana" by Yogis) which accounts for biochemical and physiological systems, seems to require and strengthen a more human connection between practitioner and patient in the healing encounter.[31]

Alternative treatments tend to use natural products and to stress the role of nutrition in wellness and prevention. They are distinguished from mainstream medicine by their emphasis on the "subjective experience" of the patient and by their insistence that therapists should focus on the person rather than just on the disease.[32]

It isn't just a new philosophical approach that has promoted a resurgence in alternative medicine, however. In places where orthodox medical care was not readily available to a large section of the population, marginal practices have emerged to fill the gap.[33] More recently, a second major reason frequently cited as responsible for public disillusionment with the present medical system is the injuries that stem from medical interventions and drugs that are supposed to cure but in fact exacerbate the problems (called "iatrogenic disease").[34]

We'd be the first to admit that unfortunately there is still a great deal of quackery in the field of alternative medicine. Many "New Age" remedies have no measurable impact, and, of course, no supporting research. Some charlatans notwithstanding, however, many alternative medical approaches are ethical and justified, and this fact is being rapidly accepted by consumers and their physicians alike. As *Time* magazine announced in a fall 1996 special report, "the alternative movement has progressed from offbeat practitioners and adventurous patients to the medical establishment itself."

The National Institutes of Health have established an Office of Alternative Medicine, with 10 federally funded, reputable centers throughout the country devoted to evaluating promising unconventional treatments. Stanford University's Center for Research in Disease Prevention is one of them. Another is the Center for Alternative Medicine Research at Boston's Beth Israel Hospital, which is associated with Harvard University. This general upgrading of attitudes toward alternative medicines is rapidly forcing even very conservative doctors to at least consider what's going on elsewhere in the world.

THE FDA RULES THE ROOST

The United States Food and Drug Administration (FDA) will allow no health claims to be made for Cernitin, or, for that matter, any other products that have not been exhaustively researched for efficacy and long-term safety in the United States.

This research costs an average of $100 million per product to meet FDA regulations. For most nutritional supplement companies this is prohibitively expensive. Additionally, Cernitin cannot be patent protected by any company doing the research and development, so a competitor could immediately bring the same product to market but without any research and development costs to recoup. The result is a built-in limitation on the health claims that can be made for Cernitin in the United States. This limitation on health claims also tends to discourage companies who depend on advertising to get their point across.

Companies now making prescription drugs have considerably more governmental clout and marketing muscle to support them than smaller, privately held companies seeking to launch alternative products, such as Cernitin. Once an alternative natural product has been discovered, what drug companies will do if they are interested in the results is to put major funding toward research geared to identifying and isolating aspects of the natural compound so they can create man-made substitutes that can be patented.

THE CONCLUSION: IT WORKS!

We hope we've convinced you that flower pollen extract is a safe, natural, and effective way to treat the symptoms of one of man's most troubling conditions: BPH. You probably know more now about the amazing discovery and scientific inquiry into Cernitin than many people know about the drugs they commonly take every day. Remember that knowledge is power, and by knowing as much as possible about this revolutionary treatment you can take charge of your body and your health.

We've also shown you how even the most promising drugs and therapies can be thwarted by the FDA. Just because you haven't heard of something doesn't necessarily mean that it doesn't work—it could just mean that the manufacturer isn't permitted to tell you about its benefits in clear and understandable terms. That's why we embarked on the journey of writing this book. We felt that men, especially older men, were entitled to this information so as to be able to decide for themselves which route to take in treating the symptoms of BPH.

5

THE PROSTATE CURE:
A SEVEN-STEP PROACTIVE PROGRAM

How should a man choose a physician for his BPH?

*

Which is better, a primary care physician or a urologist?

*

What else does a man need to do to encourage prostate health?

*

What is the relationship between depression and BPH?

While Cernitin on its own works to treat BPH, its degree of success may vary among men who use it. For those for whom Cernitin has limited success, as well as those who experience dramatic relief, it is still only the beginning of a practical program to maximize your ability to regain and maintain your health. There remain a number things that you must do to enhance the effectiveness of Cernitin and to improve your overall health. Here are the seven steps in The Prostate Cure program that will help you:

1. *Select and work with a physician for a proper diagnosis.*
2. *Take Cernitin to reduce your symptoms.*
3. *Exercise regularly for total health maintenance.*

4. *Maintain your ideal body weight.*

5. *Eat a diet healthful for proper functioning of the urinary tract.*

6. *Fight anxiety, depression, and stress.*

7. *Take yourself lightly.*

Let's look at each of these seven steps separately.

STEP 1: SELECT AND WORK WITH A PHYSICIAN FOR A PROPER DIAGNOSIS

According to Dr. Leo Galland, a New York doctor in private practice who specializes in treating undiagnosed and difficult-to-treat illnesses, your medical treatment will be more effective if you have good rapport and communication with your doctor. He suggests, therefore, that you state your needs clearly and firmly, and feel good about doing so, remembering that the doctor isn't there to "cure" you, but rather to help your body heal itself.

Before you see your doctor, define what you want to get out of a visit. Make a list of questions you want answered (remember, we said in Chapter 2 that as you read through this book, you might want to jot down a list of specific questions) and fax it to the doctor. To be on the safe side, bring a second copy of the list with you when you see the doctor.[1]

The physician you choose to help you take control of your BPH will likely be either a primary care physician—especially if you are in a managed care health plan—or a urologist to whom your primary physician will refer you. As we indicated in Chapter 2, either doctor may order a variety of tests, but before ordering any tests, he will first obtain your medical history. This process will probably begin by his simply asking you why you've come to him. Physicians call this the "chief complaint."

From this point on, he will be asking a number of questions to help him distinguish between BPH and the other disorders we discussed in Chapter 1 (such as prostatitis, prostatodynia, and prostate cancer) that have the same or similar symptoms. Certainly your doctor will want to know where you experience pain or discomfort, when it occurs, and how frequently.

He may ask a lot of other personal questions that many men find hard to answer or embarrassing because they don't talk about these situations easily. Rest assured, your doctor is not simply invading your privacy. Think of him as a detective attempting to hone his initial impression and to narrow down the medical culprit.

He will want to know about your health in general and, likely, about your sex life. He may ask these questions directly or may refer to a health questionnaire that you filled out before seeing him in order to clarify or elaborate on your responses. As he gets closer to thinking your disorder is BPH, he will ask you a number of more direct questions to determine the extent that you have the symptoms we listed in Chapter 1. All the while the doctor will be sorting out your responses to exclude scarring in your urethra, abnormal contraction in your bladder neck, and nerve damage to your bladder, conditions that can have some but not all of the same symptoms as BPH.[2]

Then comes the physical exam. The extent of the examination likely depends on whether your doctor is your primary care physician or a urologist. If he is a primary care physician, and this is the first time that you have visited him, he may do a complete physical examination. If he is a urologist, he will be more likely to focus his examination on the genitourinary tract.[3] Of course, whichever doctor you are with, he will do the exam that many men despise, the digital rectal exam (DRE). Before or after that exam, he may order one or more of the tests we have indicated at the beginning of Chapter 2.

If your primary physician refers you to a urologist to rule out prostate cancer, and it is determined that you do not have prostate cancer, then it may well be the primary care physician who will have the major responsibility for continuing to monitor your BPH, dependent in part on how your insurance plan works.

A survey of 344 primary care physicians attending various scientific meetings in 1995 indicated that while the primary care physicians surveyed are playing an increasing role in the diagnosis and management of prostate disorders, they were not taking full advantage of clinical practice guidelines of the American Urological Association. Only 38 percent of the physicians indicated they used the American Urological Association's symptom score in their practice—although 61 percent did indicate they were aware of it.

The same survey also showed that the most popular BPH therapies that primary care physicians used were watchful waiting and long-acting alpha blockers.[4] If these therapies suit you—and they may be all that many men need—then you may be happy to remain in the care of your primary physician. If you need to feel more confident about your physician's treatment or care, then you may also want to at least consult a urologist before you return to the treatment plan of your primary physician, or you may desire to follow the guidelines of the urologist.

When you discuss *your* treatment options for BPH with your doctor, make sure you understand what's happening to you and what your doctor thinks your options are—even though you may not agree in the long run. But you can't really disagree until you fully understand what your doctor is saying. It's his job to explain what's happening to you in such a way that you *can* understand it.

Remember, however, that your doctor can only present you with choices; he cannot decide for you, nor should he. You alone can

> *The more you know, and the more you understand about your particular situation, the better equipped you will be to make appropriate choices in conjunction with your physician.*

make the decision as to whether the discomfort or inconvenience you experience is sufficient to warrant surgery—even though you may have a long way to go before it is an emergency situation—or whether you can get along for at least a while by taking medication or trying natural remedies. You are not the obedient child of your doctor; you are working in partnership with him for your best health.

If you decide to have surgery, or your situation is so problematic that you can no longer accept alternative treatments, do not choose a surgeon until you have studied his credentials. Even if you are limited to the doctors in your health management program, there is still more than one doctor you can select from, and some choices you can make. You can contact the American Medical Association at (312) 464-5000 to get a professional profile of your physician, including where he or she trained. To verify that your physician has passed the specialty board examinations, contact the American Board of Medical Specialties at (847) 491-9091.

Talk to those doctors in whom you are interested about your concerns and your fears. We know that's easier said than done, but don't be afraid to appear ignorant, and don't get sidetracked by the feeling that the questions you ask are dumb or that the doctor thinks you're being silly. Good doctors won't think this way; and for the most part, if you want to know, they want you to know.

Ask the surgeon you are considering how many times he has successfully performed the surgery or procedure you are considering. Your surgery will likely go better and you will feel more comfortable if you find a surgeon who performs that type of surgery or procedure every day or several days a week.[5]

If you don't like the way the doctor interacts with you or the manner in which he gives you information about your condition or his experience, by all means seek another doctor. You will do better with your recovery if you have confidence in your surgeon, in terms of both his skill and his personal interaction with you, because you are going to have to see this guy more than once.

Neil Fiore, a psychologist practicing today in Berkeley, California, who was diagnosed 24 years ago with testicular cancer that had metastasized, is a strong patient advocate. Dr. Fiore says that patients whose doctors consider them "hard to deal with" tend to live longer than patients who are overly deferential to their doctors.[6] Now, we're not advocating that you set out to deliberately antagonize your doctor, but we are telling you that your whole treatment plan will work better if you are well-informed and take an active (some would say aggressive) part in your treatment and recovery decisions.

STEP 2: TAKE CERNITIN TO REDUCE YOUR SYMPTOMS

Cernitin, of course, is at the heart of the man's cure. For maximum effectiveness, we recommend you take at least two 63 mg Cernitin tablets twice a day. This is the amount that has been used in all clinical studies, and it seems to be the most effective at treating the symptoms of BPH.

As we discussed at length in the previous chapter, Cernitin has proven its effectiveness again and again in research studies. It is a safe and natural nutritional supplement that provides relief to many men suffering from the annoying symptoms of BPH. Significantly, it is without the drawbacks of many other treatments—the invasiveness, danger, and recovery from surgery, and the negative side effects of many prescription drugs.

STEP 3: EXERCISE REGULARLY
FOR TOTAL HEALTH MAINTENANCE

Exercise has so many general health benefits that it's hard to keep track of all of them. Dr. James Rippe, Director of the Center for Clinical and Lifestyle Research in Shrewsbury, Massachusetts, calls exercise "the closest thing to a magic bullet that exists in modern medicine."[7]

Although there is no specific exercise program that can prevent BPH, we do know that if you are exercising, you are increasing your overall general health and boosting your immune system. Regular exercise makes it easier to fight off all kinds of health problems, including prostate problems.

Exercise burns calories, helping to control weight. It lowers the risk of heart disease and cancer, and boosts strength—no matter what your age—while reducing your cholesterol level, and keeping your bones strong and joints flexible. It also helps to reverse the lowered basal metabolic rate that most people think comes naturally

Morning workouts burn more fat than those performed in the afternoon because after an all-night fast, two-thirds of the calories burned come from stores of fat. In the afternoon, the most recent meal's carbohydrates provide the main energy source, while less than half of the calories come from stored fat.[8]

with aging, but which in fact is almost wholly caused by a loss of muscle mass, which is also reversed by exercise.[9]

FITNESS INVOLVES MORE THAN JUST EXERCISE ALONE

Most fitness experts consider fitness as involving the key components of aerobic endurance, muscular strength, muscular endurance, flexibility, and body composition: A good fitness program strives to attain a balance between all of them. *Aerobic endurance* is the body's ability to exercise whole muscle groups over an extended period of time at moderate intensity. *Muscular strength* is, of course, the capacity of your body's muscles to exert a certain amount of force, while *muscular endurance* refers to how well your muscles can maintain or repeatedly generate that force.

Flexibility—being able to stretch your muscles and the tendons and ligaments that connect muscles to your bones—decreases the risk of injury while exercising. *Body composition* is concerned with the relationship of fat, bone, and muscle in your body. Their ratio provides an overall view of your health and fitness level.

SOME DO'S AND DON'TS OF A FITNESS PROGRAM

To develop the best level of fitness for you, *do* start off moderately. As you progress, work your way *gradually* into a routine that suits you. Slow gradations not only ease your body into exercise and the demands you make on it, but they help you to avoid injury. Contrary to popular myth, running is not the best exercise to get fit, because there is no one "best" exercise.

Don't keep up the same old thing over and over if it's boring for you. *Do* have fun. One of the quickest ways to avoid exercising is to

> *The important thing for long-term exercise is to find*
> *ways of getting fit that you enjoy.*

develop a workout that bores you. Adding new exercises to your workout, or changing activities, can break the monotony and add interest to your routine.

If motivation is a problem for you, *do* find a workout partner with abilities equal to your own. In this way you can encourage each other and won't be disappointed in your partner's abilities because they exceed yours.

Do stagger the intensity of your workouts and alternate by days the type of exercise you do. Leave at least one day between muscle-building exercises. Rest and alternating workouts allow your body time to recover and grow, help build endurance, and prevent injury.

Don't dehydrate yourself while exercising. During exercise the body needs four to eight ounces of water every 20 minutes to replace water loss. If you become thirsty during a workout, you've already passed out of a "safe" stage of hydration; take fluids immediately. *Do* avoid caffeine or alcohol when exercising, as both can dehydrate your body.

AEROBIC ENDURANCE

In general, walking is the simplest, and often the easiest, exercise we can do to promote health benefits. According to Dr. Rippe, nine out of 10 doctors believe that walking is the best form of exercise.[10] Walking often helps relieve prostate problem symptoms, and fast walking is an inexpensive and effective cardiopulmonary exercise.

For the best cardiopulmonary effects, the absolute *minimal* amount of walking, using the treadmill, or engaging in some other aerobic activity is 20 minutes a day, three to four days a week. Most doctors recommend 30 to 40 minutes a day, five days a week, as a minimum for an *overall* exercise program with lasting effects.

Aerobic exercise is determined by any activity that raises your pulse rate to between 50 and 75 percent of your maximum number of beats per minute. To compute your maximum number of heartbeats per minute, subtract your age from 220. Find the 50 (minimum) and 75 percent (maximum) numbers, and exercise within that range.

The Centers for Disease Control and Prevention (CDC) advise a daily activity schedule of at least 30 minutes of "moderate" activity, which is considered less physically taxing than aerobic exercise. The CDC defines "moderate" as exercise performed at an intensity of three to six METS, a physiological measure of metabolic weight. Three to six METS are roughly equivalent to walking at a rate of three to four miles an hour, whereas aerobic walking would require a more rapid pace.

The change in guidelines occurred after surveys revealed that only a fraction of Americans were still getting the recommended level of aerobic exercise, and after observational studies indicated that regular moderate exercise also appears to control weight and to reduce the risk of cardiovascular disease, osteoporosis, certain cancers, depression and anxiety disorders.[11]

Running and jogging are certainly aerobic activities, but, in addition to walking, some of the best aerobic activities are swimming, bicycling, using the treadmill, or any other exercise routine that produces a comparable increase in heart rate. You might want to vary your routine to keep from getting bored—though some men are comfortable with the consistency of a routine that they have found works for them.

If you are a stranger to aerobic exercise—
or any exercise for that matter—begin by gradually
building up your aerobic ability. Don't just jump
in the water or onto the treadmill and think that's
all there is to it. Your naivete or your
eagerness can result in injury.

While aerobic exercise can assist in weight loss, this is not its major contribution to good health. Suitable, regular exercise provides a whole range of major benefits to the body's various systems. Although your heart rate initially increases when you first begin aerobic training, once the heart is aerobically conditioned, it works more efficiently, uses less oxygen at any given workload, and produces a slower resting pulse. Aerobic exercise conditions the smooth muscles of your entire cardiovascular system, as well as those in your internal organs. It causes you to sweat more readily whenever you exert yourself, not just during exercise. This positively affects your ability to control your internal body temperature, since normally that ability declines as we get older. Regular aerobic exercise also increases your total blood volume, which also will make you less likely to overheat or dehydrate in hot weather. Finally, aerobic exercise increases the levels of high-density lipoproteins (the "good" cholesterol) and strengthens the immune system.[12]

Certainly walking is the easiest, if not the most common, aerobic exercise, provided you move faster than a slow stroll through the neighborhood. Although walking may be the simplest aerobic exercise, you nevertheless need to invest in a good pair of walking shoes to cushion shock to your feet and joints. Note that walking shoes differ from typical running shoes, and are a bit stiffer.

As with any aerobic exercise, check your pulse periodically to determine if you are within your 50 to 75 percent heartbeat target zone. In time, as you become better conditioned, walk faster or exercise a little harder to move into the upper range of that zone.

It is also important to incorporate weight-bearing exercise into your overall routine to strengthen muscle and bones and to prevent bone loss that occurs with aging. This type of exercise should be preceded by gentle stretching exercises (too vigorous stretching can also injure cold muscles) to warm up the muscles and prevent muscular damage, and to enhance flexibility.

You'll perform better and with less danger of injuring cold muscles if you have a five-minute warm-up period and five-minute cool-down period before and after both aerobic and moderate exercise. Remember, however, that the more fit you are, the greater capacity your muscles have, and the longer it takes for them to warm up for full exertion.[13]

According to physical fitness experts, a cool-down period is necessary because the body can suffer from shock if you stop exercising suddenly. Sitting down and resting immediately after aerobic exercise causes the muscles to contract, with subsequent loss of flexibility and stiffness.[14]

Warm-up should consist of the same movements as your exercise program in order to slowly condition the muscles you are going to be using. So, for moderate walking or treadmill exercise, make the warm-up a slow walk. For weight-bearing exercises, gentle stretching of those muscles used in the exercises is effective.

The chart that follows should help you gradually work into a healthful exercise program. It assumes you are a sedentary person just beginning a fitness program and helps you gradually build up your routine. If you do not have the time for 60 minutes of exercise all at one time, break it up into segments. Do the aerobic workout, including the five-minute warm-up and warm-down in one setting.

Week No.	Warm-Up	Exercise in 50–70% Range	Cool-Down	Stretching	Weight-Bearing Exercise	Total Time
1	5	5	5	3	0	18
2	5	6	5	4	0	20
3	5	7	5	5	0	22
4	5	8	5	6	5	29
5	5	10	5	7	7	34
6	5	12	5	8	9	39
7	5	14	5	10	11	45
8	5	16	5	12	13	51
9	5	18	5	15	15	58
10	5	20	5	15	15	60

A Sample Exercise Routine for Prostate Health
(Times Are in Minutes)

Stretch at a later time, possibly in your office. Then gradually combine stretching with weight-bearing exercises to help you warm up the muscles you will use for the weight-bearing movements.

Always consult a doctor before starting any exercise program, especially if you are over 45 years old and/or if you have been sedentary for three months or longer.[15]

Studies related to prostate cancer specifically show that a consistent exercise regimen or an occupation that requires a lot of physical activity lessen the risk of developing prostate cancer. While it's not clear why this is so, some authorities have speculated that increased physical activity may lower the level of testosterone.[16] Another theory relates to exercise helping to control free radicals, a term most of us have heard about but few understand, except that we've been told they're bad. Yes and no. To understand them we have to go back to the basics of atoms, tiny particles which, when they combine, form molecules, the body's building blocks. Normally the electrons comprising molecules exist in pairs, but when an electron loses its partner (through pollution, ultraviolet radiation, or any normal metabolic process that consumes oxygen), that leaves a single molecule—a free radical. This highly reactive and unstable free radical will attempt to latch onto whatever it comes in contact with, in the process injuring cell membranes, causing inflammation, inducing DNA mutations, and in general causing widespread disturbances in normal cellular function. Many of the characteristics of aging (e.g., gray hair, wrinkled skin) and some diseases (arthritis, lung inflammation, cancer) result from the cellular damage called oxidation, that is caused by free radicals.

We do know that overall a regularly exercised body gives off fewer free radicals, which helps deter the tissue damage they cause, although, it is true that the body does produce free radicals during exercise, or during any metabolic activity.

While there's no way to avoid free radicals—in fact, they provide the fuel for cellular reactions—a well-exercised body, natural antioxidants made in the body, and foods high in antioxidants or antioxidant supplements can help keep them in check for maximal prostate health.

STEP 4: MAINTAIN YOUR IDEAL BODY WEIGHT

Dr. William J. Evans, director of the Nutrition, Metabolism and Exercise Laboratory at the University of Arkansas for Medical Sciences, and coauthor of *Biomarkers: The 10 Keys to Prolonging Vitality* states categorically that Americans carry too much body fat and too little muscle. Rather than simply encouraging people to lose weight, he advocates changing the ratio of muscle to fat; that is, con-

> *Moderately overweight men have more than double the risk of developing prostate cancer, while those who are truly obese are four times more likely to do so.*

centrating on building muscle as a means of maintaining appropriate body weight, because people with high ratios of muscle to fat have higher metabolic rates and don't have to worry a lot about gaining weight.[17] A healthy male's body should be approximately 12 to 18 percent fat.

Although you do want to maintain some body fat because it stores energy and helps maintain body temperature, all evidence points to the fact that being overweight increases your risk of developing any cancer, including prostate cancer. One study conducted at Loma Linda University showed that obese men were twice as likely to have fatal prostate cancer than men closer to their desirable weight.[18]

Chinese researchers at Beijing Medical University have definitely linked the increase of BPH in China to an increase in the daily intake of total calories—leading to an increase in weight—as well as to the consumption of more fatty foods and animal protein, and the decreased daily intake of vegetables and whole grain.[19]

STEP 5: EAT A DIET HEALTHFUL FOR PROPER FUNCTIONING OF THE URINARY TRACT

One of the most important things you can do to reduce discomfort with BPH is to eat in such a way that you don't cause or contribute to nutritional problems. Your body needs many different nutrients just to survive in a healthy fashion, but certain foods can help reduce or prevent the exacerbation of symptoms. In Chapter 6, we present extensive dietary guidelines to help you properly fuel your body and enhance overall immunity, one of the main goals in "natural" healing.

STEP 6: FIGHT ANXIETY, DEPRESSION, AND STRESS

A major problem for many BPH sufferers is that the pain, sexual dysfunction, and embarrassment they endure can cause them to sink under a gray cloud of depression. Combine this with the stress, anxiety, and worry that accompany the symptoms of BPH as well as the relationship problems that may ensue, and you can certainly see that men with BPH are ripe for negative feelings and lowered self-esteem. Further, a negative attitude and feelings of depression can lower the defense level of your immune system and prevent healthy recovery.

While we can't always control events that happen to us, we have a great deal of control over our response to these events, and we *can* reduce their negative impact. Emotional stress is a warning signal that needs to be recognized and heeded. It is your body's way of telling you that you have too much to handle, or you're letting the little things bother you too much.[20] Either way, it says: "You need to make some kind of change." Fortunately, there are a number of things you can do to feel better about yourself and your condition.

WATCH YOUR STRESS LEVEL

If you are an individual with a high level of stress, you certainly will profit from learning some relaxation exercises and/or purchasing some relaxation tapes.

Be aware that you may come face-to-face with some of your old family or cultural rules that say relaxation is not something you can do and enjoy every day. Our society constantly informs us that relaxation is something we need to postpone until our next vacation, time off, or even until retirement.

The symptoms of BPH often leave a man feeling "out of control," which, if you are a person who always needs to feel in control, will add a considerable amount of anxiety to your life. Realize that you simply can't control the physical symptoms of BPH the way you can control your actions in job-related and recreational activities.

Few experiences are totally negative; you might reduce your stress level by asking yourself, "What awareness can BPH teach me about my need for control?" Your answers may help you to redefine your concept of "control" (much of it is illusory, or functions to help us feel more comfortable and less anxious), or to react more positively to the real control you do have. The corollary to this is to consider things you *can* do to help yourself feel more in control; for instance, to inform yourself of everything you can about BPH and the options available to you, so you can make intelligent decisions and set priorities regarding your health care. You have already taken a step along that pathway by purchasing this book and using the ideas in it.

DON'T PUT RELAXATION OFF

There are lots of little "relaxation breaks" that you can schedule into each day. They can be as simple as putting your feet up on your desk for five minutes; stopping what you are doing to breathe deeply; or instead of fuming because you're stopped at a red light, taking a couple of deep breaths. As you inhale, say to yourself, "Relax." As you exhale, say to yourself, "Let go."

Go outside for a 5- or 10-minute walk. While you are outdoors, don't forget to notice the colors of the world and how beautiful they are; how they blend together or contrast with each other; or how they're changing during the season. We know you've heard it before, but it's true: Take time to smell the roses. If you can't do it any other way, get your doctor to write a prescription for you: "Smell roses, three times daily."

CERTAIN KINDS OF MUSIC ARE GREAT STRESS-BUSTERS

Sorry, but we're not talking about rock 'n' roll here. Classical music works well for some people, enveloping them so they can "flow" with the music and think of nothing else. Soothing, relaxing music that is not familiar has been shown to affect physiological responses related to emotionality for anxious persons,[21] and to reduce the disruptive behavior of psychiatric patients during the dinner hour.[22]

Composer Steven Halpern has embraced a new vision of music and sees it as a vehicle for self-empowerment and spiritual well-being. Many people are soothed by Halpern's music immediately, although they are unable to say exactly why. Perhaps that's why some people describe it as "twentieth-century healing music."

Halpern, who today has more than 50 albums to his credit,[23] began researching the effects of his music by first playing it in waiting rooms and recovery wards in health clinics and hospitals. Babies stopped crying; patients calmed down. Quite simply, it is music that touches us at a "cellular level."

EXAMINE YOUR THINKING STYLE

Positive thinking is one of the most important things you can do to feel better emotionally. Psychologists now know that negative thinking does not arise from negative feelings, but the other way around.

The negative things you say about yourself and your condition definitely influence the way you feel during the day. The truth is that the thoughts, words, and images you experience daily can have very real positive or negative consequences on your body. Your brain often cannot distinguish whether you are imagining something or actually experiencing it.[24]

Many, if not most of us, experience at some time or another negative or erroneous thoughts that produce stress. Changing negative thoughts into more helpful, positive thoughts is called cognitive therapy. It may require close monitoring or attention to catch your negative thoughts—many of which have likely become such a part of your life that they are automatic—and active work to replace them with more positive ones.

Well-known cognitive therapists like Drs. Aaron Beck[25] and David Burns[26] have identified at least 10 common ways that we distort our thinking so that we end up feeling bad. We list them below to help you begin to reorganize your perception of your life and your disorder. Not everyone uses all 10, but don't be surprised if you spot some of your favorites in the list, although you may never have thought of them as simply "habitual ways of thinking."

TEN COMMON COGNITIVE DISTORTIONS IN THINKING

1. **Polarized (All-or-Nothing) Thinking.** You tend to see things in black and white, dividing problems and choices into two categories only. If your performance is not totally perfect, you are a total failure. What is happening to you is either "good" or "bad." Something is either possible or impossible, with no in-between. Example: There are no other options; your medical experience is certainly not going to lead to more positive experiences. In truth,

nothing is either totally good or totally bad. We never know what positive benefits a seemingly negative one can have in the future.

2. **Overgeneralization.** One of the most troublesome and most difficult-to-change distortions in the thinking process involves seeing a single negative event as a typical, never-ending pattern. Good clues to overgeneralized thinking are using all-or-nothing words such as "always," "never," "all," "every," and "none," and making absolutist statements ("This *always* happens to me." "Things *never* go right for me.").

3. **Mental Filter.** If you pick out a single negative detail and dwell on it exclusively, you're using this type of distorted thinking. The one detail is the only thing that matters, the only thing that influences your condition, your health, your future. Example: "I have BPH; I'm flawed and have lost control of my future."

4. **Disqualifying or Discounting the Positive.** Positive experiences "don't count" at all or certainly don't carry the same emotional weight as negative conditions.

5. **Jumping to Conclusions.** Making a negative interpretation even though you have no observable or known facts to support your interpretation. In order to maintain this position, you also have to *not* check things out to ascertain whether your conclusion is correct. You just "know" your position or interpretation is correct, and that's all there is to it.

6. **Catastrophizing.** Exaggerating the importance of things or the severity of a particular event and its consequences. ("BPH is the most disastrous thing that has ever happened to me. I will never recover.") Catastrophic thinking is frequently

subtly embedded in hidden fears that lead to anger. Albert Ellis, founder of rational-emotive therapy, identifies a similar cognitive distortion that he calls "awfulizing"—categorizing some happening as terrible when, in reality, its implications are only mild or moderate.

7. **Subjective Reasoning.** Here you assume that your negative emotions (or any other strong emotions, for that matter) necessarily reflect the way things truly are in the real world. ("This is the way I feel; therefore, it must be true.") A corollary to this is the belief that if you have a negative emotion, someone else is responsible for it. ("My doctor makes me feel so angry." "If I feel anxious, it is because my boss is not cooperating with me.")

8. **"Should" Statements.** These are a big trap for many people. You try to whip yourself into shape with absolute "shoulds," and if you fail, you experience guilt and, maybe, shame. It was psychoanalyst Karen Horney who introduced the concept of the "tyranny of the shoulds," wherein we make unreasonable claims and demands based on an assumed right and become angry—often enraged—with others, the world, fate, or God when our demands are thwarted or unmet. ("People should treat me better." "It's not fair that I have this disorder.") "Shoulds" and "oughts" make you feel more responsible, and therefore more guilty, than is realistic for many medical situations, especially BPH.

9. **Labeling and Mislabeling.** This is describing an event—or your own or someone else's behavior—with negative labels. Instead of accepting that we all make mistakes and that they are a learning experience, you call yourself a "loser" or a "failure."

> 10. **Personalization.** Viewing yourself as the cause of some
>   negative external event whereas in reality you were not pri-
>   marily responsible for the event. Another aspect of person-
>   alization involves believing that the actions of another—or
>   many others—are personally, and malevolently or nega-
>   tively, directed at you. Certainly, you feel, those others can
>   have no other motivation or reason for their behavior.

Remember, changing your thinking alters your reaction to stress—and stressed is "desserts" spelled backwards. Figure it out.

DON'T DWELL ON THE QUESTION, "WHY IS THIS HAPPENING TO ME?"

We know this is a question you will invariably ask yourself at first, and we know that it's equally tempting to dwell on that question with the hope that you can find some satisfactory answer. You probably won't.

A more productive and less negative approach is the one that Dr. Neil Fiore took when he was diagnosed with cancer.[27] The question he focused on was "Now that I have cancer (BPH, in your case), where do I go from here?" Rather than leave you in a stalemate as the "why me?" question does, the "what do I do now?" question mobilizes you to take whatever steps are necessary to cope with BPH and to find the appropriate treatment *for you.*

CHANGE YOUR VIEW OF EVERYDAY EXASPERATIONS OR AGGRAVATIONS

If you need help keeping in check those daily, pesky things that provoke your anger or leave you "climbing the wall," consider taking to heart the messages in psychologist Richard Carlson's book *Don't Sweat the Small Stuff . . . and It's All Small Stuff.*[28]

Dr. Carlson is a stress consultant and an expert in helping people to stop overreacting (remember "catastrophizing" from the table above?) and to transform their anxious or angry views about what's happening around them into more reassuring, positive experiences. It is the change from believing that everything is a "GREAT BIG DEAL" to reacting in a more accepting way and developing new habits of perspective.

For instance, when a stranger in an automobile cuts in front of you, rather than fuming with anger and feeling justified in doing so (a practice that raises blood pressure and stress levels and reduces immunity), Carlson suggests that we "allow the driver to have his accident somewhere else" and avoid taking personally whatever problems the driver is having.[29]

Carlson's book lists a number of exercises and techniques, including becoming aware of our moods—which, as he says, are "always on the run"—and not allowing ourselves to be fooled by the low ones. This is particularly important for men with prostate conditions, who have a tendency to think the problem is the first step to the end of sexual life.

Carlson cautions that bad or negative moods can be deceptive, often tricking us into believing that our life is worse than it really is. Question your judgment, Carlson says, and don't take your low moods too seriously. Remind yourself that a low or bad mood is an unavoidable part of being human and that it will pass. Certainly when you're experiencing a low mood, as you might be soon after a diagnosis of BPH or prostate cancer, that is not the time to analyze your life. To do so is emotional suicide, Carlson says. Wait until you're feeling better and have a more expanded perspective.[30]

STEP 7: TAKE YOURSELF LIGHTLY

Humor can be emotionally liberating. It is one of the most excellent coping mechanisms we humans have,[31] and may help men with prostate problems get through, or come out of, low periods. Widely credited for its positive physiological and psychological effects, humor reduces stress, anxiety, worry, and frustration.[32] Listen to how comedians make fun of their own prostate problems. Humor helps them, as well as the rest of us, take the sting out of our difficulties and not take our selves so seriously. It gives us that expanded perspective Dr. Carlson writes about.

Studying the effects of humor on physiology is known scientifically as "gelotology" (we never claimed that scientists have a sense of humor).[33] In spite of its unfunny name, studies of humor have shown it to raise the threshold of pain a person can experience[34] and to decrease depression.[35] One hypothesis for this is that laughter stimulates the secretion of beta-endorphins (the body's natural opiates) in the brain, thus affecting pain receptor sites on nerve cells and reducing pain sensations.[36] As early as the thirteenth century, medical treatises depicted laughter as an anesthetic for surgical procedures.[37]

The use of humor is touted in such fields as business and management, because the changed perspective and attitude it induces facilitates creative problem solving.[38] Humor allows us to relax some of the organizational or societal confines in which we regularly operate, thereby permitting us to see connections we might not otherwise see.[39] So, to keep your mind and body lively, don't develop what psychologist Daniel O. Dugan has termed "psychosclerosis," the loss of a humorous perspective toward life, or, more specifically, the "hardening of attitudes."[40]

Laughter, which requires the coordinated movement of 15 facial muscles,[41] releases excessive physical and psychological energy, resulting in a mood-elevating and relaxing effect. Technically it causes spasmodic skeletal muscle contractions (with subsequent relaxation), rapid heartbeat, and changes in breathing. By aiding ventilation and clearing mucus, laughter helps the breathing pattern of many persons with chronic respiratory conditions, such as emphysema.[42] Dr. W. J. Fry, Jr., a medical doctor who has done research on the effects of laughter and humor for more than 30 years, believes that laughing 100 times a day is equal to 10 minutes of rowing.[43]

Although laughter is considered a form of stress, it is beneficial stress or "eustress" because it does not produce an increase in common "stress hormones," and because laughter is followed by systemic relaxation. In fact, after a good, hearty laugh, people feel "pleasantly drained."[44]

When 39 young college women watched a 28-minute segment of a Bill Cosby routine, the amount of secretory immunoglobulin A (S-Ig-A) in their saliva increased significantly (S-Ig-A is an antibody found in saliva that protects against respiratory and gastrointestinal tract infections). The researchers discovered, however, that the healing effects of humor on the immune system don't necessarily require even a smile. The women's immunity levels improved with exposure, regardless of whether they expressed overt laughter.[45]

The general public could no longer ignore the healing aspects of humor after the 1979 publication of Norman Cousins's book *Anatomy of an Illness as Perceived by the Patient: Reflections on Healing.*[46] In the book he describes his remarkable recovery from a rare and serious arthritic disease (seronegative spondyloarthropathy), thanks in large part to a supportive doctor who allowed him to leave the hospital on weekends to view reruns from the television series *Candid Camera* and funny, slapstick movies (e.g., Marx Brothers comedies). Among the results were hours of pain-free sleep and decreased paralysis.

The productions that tickled Cousin's funny bone may not necessarily do the same for everyone, however. A limited study of a
humor program with older adults living in an apartment complex in
West Virginia showed that this particular group preferred a live pup-
pet show and the entertainment provided by a live comedian over
viewing funny television episodes and movies.[47]

Whatever your own preferences, don't ignore laugh-provoking
situations. Exercise your sense of humor just as regularly as you do
your physical body to avoid getting caught in a rut of negative attitudes and self-perception. Not taking yourself so seriously helps you
face the future with a more positive, and certainly quite different,
perception.

CREATE YOUR OWN "MIRTH-AID KIT."[48]

Develop a library of humorous resources. If you don't know already
what makes you laugh, explore and learn. The appreciation of
humor can be learned. It is an intuitive intelligence that can be nour-
ished if you're willing.[49]

If cultivating humor is new to you, head for your public library.
We went to ours and simply looked up "humor." We found 319
subtopics, with 1,158 entries of humorous books, and we didn't even
make a stab at searching the videotape selections. You may also wish
to consult the American Association for Therapeutic Humor or visit
their website.[50]

Begin to keep on hand cartoons that make you chuckle, silly
songs, lightweight books, audio or video tapes that make you laugh,
and wacky television shows—whatever makes *you* laugh—to draw
on when you're feeling negative or down. One man we know buys
cartoon books that reliably make him laugh, but instead of reading

them as soon as he gets them, he puts them aside for those days when he needs a laugh lift. You may not immediately fill your life with gales of laughter, but by gradually inserting a few more snickers and giggles into each day, you're paving the road to joy . . . and better health.

6

LIVING WELL IS THE BEST REVENGE

*How do weight, diet, and exercise influence
the health of the prostate?*

*

How much trouble does a high-fat diet cause?

*

What are essential fatty acids (EFAs) and what role do they play?

*

How does selenium affect the prostate?

*

Should I drink less liquid to help control my symptoms?

*

What liquids are best?

*

Will vitamins help?

*

Can I take too many vitamins?

C ertainly it has been well established in the popular literature
that diet and lifestyle changes can make a difference in
certain medical conditions. One of the earliest men to
write about this was Norman Cousins, who helped heal a rare and
extremely painful collagen disease with laughter (as described in the
preceding chapter) and high doses of Vitamin C.[1]

The autopsy of Nathan Pritikin, creator of the severely restricting program for reducing or reversing heart disease, showed that his arteries were those of a 30-year-old man, although Pritikin was in his 50s when he died. Dr. Dean Ornish's programs and popular books indicate that persons with heart disease can often avoid surgery and reverse their disease with a combination of a low-fat (10 percent) diet, regular exercise, and meditation. As early as 1971 the United States Department of Agriculture was saying that dramatic potential savings from major health problems would take place if diets could be improved.

When the well-known newsletter *Bottom Line Personal* asked three of the nation's top doctors—one each in their fourth, fifth and sixth decade, and each in good health—to share the health issues they personally face today, they all indicated that the interrelationships between weight, diet, exercise, and stress, and their effects on illness, were of critical importance. As their first line of defense against vulnerability to disease, all three physicians indicated that they watch their weight, exercise regularly (varying from three or four times a week to daily) to stay fit and reduce stress, and maintain healthy diets rich in fruits, vegetables, whole grains, and fish, and low in saturated fats. One of them, Dr. Bernadine Healy, former director of the National Institutes of Health, also indicated that she took a multivitamin—supplemented with key antioxidants (Vitamins C and E), because they have been shown to boost the immune system—plus calcium, to combat bone loss. All three doctors indicated that attitude was equally as important to their well-being, stress being critically related to lowered immunity. They believe that by remaining positive and optimistic, and by focusing not on their vulnerabilities but rather on how they can prevent disease in general, they are better able to find activities that are fun and fulfilling.[2]

Much of the information we have for using lifestyle changes to affect BPH comes from studies of the correlation of diet and lifestyle with prostate cancer. However, a few studies have also been conducted regarding the relationship between diet and BPH, and undoubtedly more will be done in the future. In general, they show that a low-fat diet, the consumption of more fish and less red meat, and the inclusion of more fruits and vegetables contributes significantly to prostate health as well as to overall health. The more vegetables the better, since vegetables add dietary fiber and antioxidant nutrients. Less meat and more vegetables reduces the amount of circulating hormones in the body, decreasing the risk of both BPH and prostate cancer.

A 1982 report by the National Research Council named prostate cancer as one of three forms of cancer (along with breast and colon cancers) most strongly linked to dietary factors.[3] Cancer deaths in 32 countries have been linked to the consumption of animal fat.[4] In 1909, the average person in the United States consumed about 125 grams of fat per day. Today the consumption is closer to 175 grams. Shortening, margarine, refined salad oils, and cooking oils account for about 50 percent of that amount. Fat is the common name for what scientists and doctors call lipids and triglycerides. It has been associated consistently with prostate cancer risk and is definitely a major culprit.[5]

> *Fortunately, a diet designed to promote prostate health and prevent prostate cancer is an overall healthy diet that will also reduce a man's risk of heart attack or stroke. While diet factors alone probably aren't enough to cause prostate cancer, there are some dietary changes men can make to reduce their risks.*

IS THERE TOO MUCH OF A GOOD THING
WITH VITAMIN SUPPLEMENTS?

Put simply, the answer to the above question is, "Yes." Before we talk about dietary changes, we want to caution you that, for the most part, it is best to get your vitamins from the food you eat. We realize, however, that many people eat a diet that does not allow them to get all the vitamins they need, and therefore they choose to take supplements. Taking a multivitamin daily probably will not hurt you, but getting too much of certain vitamins can be worse than getting too little. For instance, persons on anticoagulant (blood-thinning) medication should avoid high doses of Vitamin E, because it can result in prolonged bleeding.

Vitamins are categorized as fat-soluble (dissolve more readily in oil) and water-soluble (dissolve readily in water). The water-soluble vitamins of the B complex and C are, for the most part, excreted in the urine; thus there is small risk of accumulating too much within the body. The excretion process takes several hours, however, and doses several times higher than the Reference Daily Intake (RDI) can have toxic effects. Long-term use of minerals such as iron, zinc, and selenium at levels somewhat over the RDI may be associated with greater risk of toxicity.

Excess amount of fat-soluble vitamins—Vitamins A, D, E, and K (supplied by intestinal bacteria)—*are not excreted* in the urine; hence, consuming high doses of these vitamins on a regular basis can lead to toxic buildup. A Japanese study showed that even a low daily intake of Vitamin A and beta-carotenes (found in orange and dark-green colored vegetables and converted into Vitamin A in the body) constituted a significant risk factor for prostatic cancer. (For more information on beta-carotenes, see the following section entitled "Eat More Salads, Fresh Vegetables and Fruits.")[7]

Although many of the studies related to vitamins and prostate

THE FUSS ABOUT RDAs

There is a great deal of misunderstanding about the term Recommended Daily Allowance (RDA) with respect to certain nutrients and whether or not they are adequate for good health. RDAs are levels that should be reached *as averages in a period of several days,* not necessarily daily. They were never meant to be guidelines for consumers, since they were initially designed to serve as standards for planning food supplies for population *groups.*

RDAs are used, however, as a partial basis for developing other guidelines that *are* intended for consumers, such as the Food Guide Pyramid, released by the United States Department of Agriculture in 1992. Generally the federal government's approach to dietary intervention does not recommend supplementing its recommended "typical" or "mainstream" diet with vitamins or nutritional supplements. This position raises serious questions for advocates of various alternative approaches to diet, who contend that the typical American diet is not sufficient to promote *optimal* health or to prevent eventual chronic illness. These advocates run the gamut from suggesting supplementing the diet somewhat beyond RDAs to supplementation using amounts well-above RDAs, to even avoiding or eliminating specific foods or types of food to treat or prevent certain conditions.[6]

To correct some of these problems, the FDA recently replaced the term Recommended Daily Allowance (RDA) with RDI, Reference Daily Intake—so you will see more of this term as RDA amounts are gradually replaced in newer publications.

difficulties have used high amounts of vitamins, these were carefully controlled studies with regard to humans, or, more frequently, laboratory studies used on animals or tissue outside the body. So, we caution you again to be especially careful not to overdose on fat-soluble vitamins by eating excessive natural amounts and/or taking more supplements than recommended.

EAT A LOW-FAT DIET

Maintaining a low-fat diet is one of the simplest things you can do for your general health, for the health of your prostate, and for giving your immune system a hearty boost.

Asian men in Japan and China who eat those countries' traditional low-fat diet of vegetables and fish have been shown to have lower incidences of prostate cancer than men who leave their Asian countries and begin to eat a diet closer to the standard high-fat American diet.

In various places in this book we talk about the effect of the Western diet on various aspects of health, and in this chapter we suggest some ways you can modify your diet. Although a relatively rare study of 20 Native Hawaiians with multiple risk factors for cardiovascular disease did not have to do specifically with prostate health, it indicated, once again, the damages caused by the typical Western diet. For 21 days, participants ate a "pre-Western-contact" (traditional) diet, which was low in fat (7 percent), high in complex carbohydrates (78 percent), with moderate protein (15 percent). Participants were encouraged to eat as much as they wanted. The study showed that Hawaiians who ate their traditional food, rather than a Western diet, had an average weight loss of approximately 17 pounds and significant reductions in serum cholesterol levels and blood pressure.[8]

One nutrition specialist suggests that the body uses animal fat to make excess sex hormones, and by reducing his intake of animal foods, a man will reduce the amount of fat available to be converted into the male hormones.[9] Some researchers have shown that a high-fat diet, low in fiber, raises the level of both testosterone and certain

> *Don't plan on eliminating all fat from your diet,*
> *because certain fats, consumed in moderate amounts,*
> *are necessary to help the body absorb certain vitamins*
> *(A, E, D and K, and beta-carotene). So cut down*
> *by being selective in the kind of fats you consume.*

estrogens that stimulate prostate growth.[10] A more likely explanation, however, is that fat intake is linked to the general fact that tumors grow more rapidly with a high-fat diet than with a low-fat diet. At least this is true for mice, according to a study conducted at Sloan-Kettering by Dr. William Fair and pharmacologist Warren Heston and reported by Leon Jaroff in a *Time* magazine article.

MEET THE OMEGA FAMILY

With respect to fat consumption, "saturated" and "unsaturated" are labels with which you need to become very familiar. Also important are the terms "essential" and "nonessential" fats, the latter being found in meats and dairy products.

Essential fatty acids (EFAs) are polyunsaturated fats that can be subdivided into the Omega-6 (linoleic acid) and Omega-3 (linolenic acid) groups. They are necessary for the regulation of many functions in the human body. Since our bodies are unable to manufacture them, they must be supplied through our diet.

Among their many healthful functions, essential fatty acids produce sex and adrenal hormones, and control cell growth—including abnormal cell growth in the prostate. Essential fatty acids are part of the outer membrane of every cell, where they protect against

The importance of maintaining adequate levels of EFAs in the body cannot be overstated, as their presence affects every aspect of our health and biological functioning. Every function of our body requires energy, and energy production begins at the cellular level where EFAs begin their beneficial activities.

viruses, bacteria, and allergens. They also help to retain proteins within the cell membrane and to regulate materials entering the cell. EFAs are crucial in the process of electron transport needed for both cellular energy and cell communication.

When the body is deficient in EFAs, it changes sugar to fat much more rapidly than normal, causing blood sugar levels to plummet. The result is that we feel hungry and irritable. EFAs help dissolve body fat into bodily fluids, decreasing blood cholesterol and triglyceride levels. They also distribute the fat-soluble vitamins A, D, E, and K throughout the body, insulate nerves, and help regulate body temperature. As if all this weren't enough, EFAs also give our immune systems a boost. In 1982 Dr. J. R. Vane shared the Nobel Prize for Medicine for his work proving how the metabolism of Omega-3 fatty acids helps to prevent heart problems.

Nutritionists believe that the proper ratio of these two EFAs is as important as the EFAs themselves, and that the optimum ratio is four parts of linolenic acid (Omega-3) to one part linoleic acid (Omega-6). The best dietary source that contains this vital ratio is flaxseed oil, the plant version of the same cholesterol-lowering Omega-3 fatty acids for which fish and fish oil are famous, making it a good alternative for people who don't like fish. Flaxseed also contains lignans, powerful antioxidants that stop cells from becoming cancerous.[12]

Omega-6 fatty acids are also found in vegetable oils, most grains, and beans. Other essential fats that exist in the Omega-3 group are found in fresh walnuts, pumpkin seeds, fish (salmon, bluefish, trout, mackerel, tuna, and sardines), and canola oil. Essential fatty acids— such as olive oil and evening primrose oil—are required by the prostate gland in order for it to perform properly. They also help reduce the amount of urine left in the bladder.

Fat consumed in the traditional Japanese diet comes from fish and the oils in soybean products, all of which contain significant amounts of the omega-3 fatty acids, which are believed to protect against heart disease and cancer. A study conducted at the University of Illinois in Urbana showed that BPH activity remained low when soybean protein and raw beef (not charcoal-broiled beef) were consumed. BPH activity was raised ninefold by charcoal-broiled beef.[13]

To help you in adhering to a low-fat diet, here are some helpful guidelines:

Select lean meats and low-fat products. Meat eaters have a two-and-a-half-times higher incidence of prostate cancer than do vegetarians,[14] but according to the Illinois study above, if you must eat beef, make it raw. Unfortunately, currently this also increases the chances of ingesting dangerous *E. coli* bacteria (remember the Jack-in-the-Box scare?), so to be on the safe side, use fowl, seafood, eggs, and low-fat dairy products for protein rather than beef.

Switch to skim milk and products made from skim milk rather than whole milk.

Give up fried foods. Bake or broil instead.

Say good-bye to fat-filled salad dressings and rich sauces. Use unsaturated fats like olive and canola oils. Dr. Isadore Rosenfeld says that men with high dietary levels of alphalinoleic acid—found in the polyunsaturated fats of meat, dairy products, and some vegetable oils—have almost three and a half times more prostate cancer.[15]

Consume more soy-based foods. Japanese and Chinese men have another diet advantage over men from other cultures. They consume a lot of food made from soybeans, such as miso soup, tofu (also known as "bean curd"), and products made from it. Because tofu is soft and porous, it will easily absorb the flavor of any dish in which it is cooked. Tofu is an excellent protein. In the United States, soy milk has become an important food for some health-minded people, and especially for those who don't like milk or don't digest it well.

Soy-based foods are high in phytochemicals and a substance called genisten, which some health-food-oriented people believe helps detoxify DHT. Genisten has estrogen-like properties, which may inhibit the growth of prostatic cancer early in its development.[16]

REDUCE YOUR CALORIC INTAKE

On the average, Japanese citizens tend to live six or seven years longer than American men and women, and some think this is due not only to the low-fat diet with more fish and soybean products but also to the fact that the Japanese consume fewer calories. In fact, they have the lowest daily caloric intake of any industrialized nation.

One good way to reduce your caloric intake is to add more fruits and vegetables to your diet, which will increase bulk and fiber and result in your feeling full faster. Don't consume empty calories such as ice cream and alcohol, while ignoring other important foods.

The eight persons who lived in the self-contained Biosphere 2 in the Arizona desert for two years were restricted to the kinds of foods they could grow, so they naturally ate more vegetables and fruits. Their food intake dropped to around 2,200 calories per day, compared to the 2,500 to 3,300 calories they were used to consuming. The result was a decrease in blood pressure, blood sugar, insulin, and cholesterol levels.[17] As you can see, reducing your calories does not mean dropping down to a starvation diet, but rather consuming less meats and more fruits, vegetables, beans, and grains, which is what we advocate throughout this chapter for both general and prostatic health.

IMPROVE YOUR SELENIUM INTAKE

Selenium is an essential trace mineral discovered in 1817 by Swedish chemist Jons Jakob Berzelius, who named it after the moon goddess Selene. Selenium originates in the soil, where it is absorbed by growing plants. In the 1950s, research into the function of selenium escalated, and it was discovered that selenium is absorbed into the molecules of an enzyme called glutathione peroxidase, which is essential for the protection of red blood cells and cell membranes. Selenium began to be recognized as an important antioxidant and cancer-preventer.

Almost half of a man's supply of selenium is concentrated in the testicles and portions of the seminal ducts adjacent to the prostate gland. A strong association between a low selenium level and the risk of developing gastrointestinal and prostatic cancers was established in a 1983 study that compared 111 subjects who developed cancer during the five years following collection of blood serum samples of selenium levels with 210 cancer-free subjects matched for age, race, sex, and smoking history.[18]

A multicenter, double-blind, randomized, placebo-controlled cancer-prevention trial conducted at seven dermatology clinics in the eastern United States with 1,312 patients found that taking 200

> *Good sources of selenium include whole-grain products, garlic, onions, shellfish, meat, chicken, mushrooms, and milk. Supplements are not recommended, as there is only a narrow margin between safe and toxic doses of selenium.*

micrograms of selenium daily did not protect against skin cancers. But it did produce significantly lower rates of total cancer incidences—including colon, prostate, and lung cancers—than for those taking placebos. The authors recommend, however, that before new public health recommendations regarding selenium supplementation can be made, their results be confirmed in an independent trial of appropriate design.[19]

Selenium tends to offset cadmium's cancer-promoting effects. While it may seem merely a cancer-preventing move to cancel the effects of this toxic trace element (found in foods grown in cadmium-polluted soil and in tobacco), at least one study has also shown that cadmium concentrations were "considerably higher" in human BPH tissue than in normal prostate tissue and "markedly increased" in cancerous tissue.[20] It has also been established that men who live in areas where the soil is rich in selenium tend to have lower rates of cancer.[21]

DRINK EIGHT GLASSES OF WATER DAILY

The natural reaction to frequent and urgent urination is usually to cut back on fluid intake; however, a man who does this runs the risk of dehydration and/or the strong possibility of developing a bladder infection. Even though persons with BPH feel like they shouldn't drink lots of water in order to control urinary symptoms, you should drink at least eight glasses of water a day. Not only is that amount necessary for good health, but it also assures that any urine retained in the bladder remains fairly diluted, reducing the risk of infection.

THE FROTH OF LIQUID JADE: GREEN TEA

After water, tea is the most popular drink in the world. Green tea, called the "froth of liquid jade" and the "elixir of life" by ancient Chinese poets,[22] is such a healthful brew that you should add it to your repertoire of disease fighters and drink, at the very least, two cups daily.

Although black, oolong, and green teas are all made from the leaf of the plant *Camellia sinenis,* green tea is the only one of the three in which the leaves are not crushed and oxidized. Instead they are steamed, which prevents oxidation, then they are rolled and dried.[23] Herb teas, of course, are not "true" teas at all, but some combination of the roots, leaves, or flowers of plants other than *Camellia sinenis,* which you may recognize by its name as a cousin of the flowering camellia bushes that grow in many gardens.

Probably the first book to tout the benefits of green tea was written in 1211 A.D. by the monk Eisai, who called it a "miraculous medicine for the maintenance of health."[24] Although the Chinese have claimed for thousands of years that tea had healthful properties, only recently have scientists been able to investigate these claims by isolating the components of tea.

Dr. Lester Mitscher, a professor of medicinal chemistry at the University of Kansas in Lawrence, advised the editors of *Bottom Line Personal* that green tea contains the strongest known disease-fighting antioxidant. Called epigallocatechin gallate, or EGCG, it is a particular kind of bioflavonoid that is 25 times more effective as an antioxidant than Vitamin E and 100 times more effective than Vitamin C, both of which are also contained in green tea.[25]

Not found in black tea or only in small amounts (5 to 10 mg per cup, compared to 40-90 mg per cup in green tea), EGCG is a member of a family of chemicals known as polyphenols, naturally occurring compounds that act as powerful antioxidants (bioflavonoids are a type of polyphenol). It works by interfering with or inhibiting the production of urokinase, an enzyme crucial for cancer growth and one of the most frequently found enzymes in human cancer.

In tests conducted at the Cancer Prevention Division of the National Cancer Center Research Institute in Tokyo, Dr. H. Fujiki and his team of researchers were able to reduce the number of tumors in animals by 73 percent using EGCG.[26]

Although the effects of EGCG specifically on humans has yet to be determined, hints of its effect were evident as early as the 1970s when epidemiologists discovered that the people living in the Shi-

THE BENEFITS OF BIOFLAVONOIDS

Sometimes called simply flavonoids, the bioflavonoids are a group of some 500 compounds found in such foods as the white part of citrus peels, in red and yellow onions, apricots, rose hips, and, of course, green tea. Once thought to be nothing more than a kind of food dye, they work in conjunction with Vitamin C to strengthen the walls of small blood vessels and capillaries, fight viruses, inhibit the actions of certain cancer promoters (carcinogens), and perform a variety of other biological activities. They are often used in foods to keep metals from oxidizing and affecting the taste of fats, oils, and salad dressings. Their prevention of oxidation is one of the things that makes them helpful in the battle against free radicals.

zouoka Prefecture in central Japan had lower death rates from all forms of cancer than those living in other areas. After careful examination of a number of factors, the only difference they could find was that the residents of Shizouoka Prefecture, where a lot of tea plants were grown, drank significantly more green tea than people living in areas with higher rates of cancer.[27]

Some researchers have speculated that at least one of the reasons why Japanese become more susceptible to prostate cancer when they emigrate to the West is the decrease in their consumption of green tea. In a laboratory study where testosterone was added to prostate cancer cells to make them grow, the addition of green tea extract caused them to grow more slowly. The more green tea, the slower the growth.[28]

Japanese researchers are beginning to accumulate evidence that drinking green tea also reduces cholesterol levels, as well as lowering triglycerides, blood pressure, and body fat in laboratory rats.[29] You should be aware, however, that these studies use high potent amounts of green tea—the equivalent for humans of anywhere from 5 to 20 cups of green tea daily. If you don't want to consume that many cups, you can increase the benefits of each single cup by adding green tea extract.[30]

EAT MORE SALADS, FRESH VEGETABLES, AND FRUITS

Many of us have been conditioned from childhood to believe that a diet rich in animal protein is healthful and hearty. Wrong! Yet, there are still men who will tell you proudly, "I'm a meat and potatoes man." The truth is that too much protein weakens the heart, speeds the deposit of fatty plaque in the arteries, reduces the effectiveness of the immune system, and promotes the formation of free radicals. Some nutrition experts believe that people who eat a low-protein diet generate more body heat, which means less body fat. The traditional Chinese diet contains about one-third less protein than Americans eat.

To reduce the amount of protein in your diet, fill up on vegetables and fruits by including five to eight servings a day. Fruits and vegetables contain phytochemicals (trace substances that protect plants), which are powerful antioxidants. Phytochemicals help to lower cholesterol, reduce blood pressure, detoxify blood, rebuild the liver, relieve the inflammation caused by allergies and arthritis, alleviate depression and impotency, and help detect and deter tumors. Happily, for a varied diet, there are tens of thousands of them found in fruits, vegetables, beans, and natural grains. One study of 122,261 men found a lower death rate from prostate cancer in men who ate green and yellow vegetables every day.[31]

Beta-carotenes are the natural pigments that create the color in dark green (kale, broccoli, spinach), orange (carrots, sweet potatoes, pumpkins), red (red peppers, tomatoes), and deep-yellow vegetables and fruits (apricots, cantaloupes, mangoes, peaches, cabbage, winter squash and Brussels sprouts). Converted to Vitamin A in the body, beta-carotenes repair damaged DNA; protect the mucous membranes of the mouth, nose, esophagus and lungs (our first line of defense against invading organisms) and cell membranes; and enrich and support the overall immune system. They are one of our major sources of carotenoids, some of the most potent plant antioxidants. Taken in general, carotenoids are a group of several kinds of pigments in fruits and vegetables and include alpha-carotene, beta-carotene, lycopene, lutein, and many other compounds that are associated with a reduced cancer risk when consumed in natural foods.

Add plenty of cruciferous vegetables (Brussels sprouts, cabbage, broccoli, cauliflower, and other members of the cabbage family) to your diet, as they contain dithiothiones—substances that eliminate the destructive properties of cancer-causing agents.[32] Broccoli and

Brussels sprouts, along with kale, carrots, and green onions also contain a potent cancer-fighting chemical called sulforaphane.[33]

Research suggests that many men who develop BPH are not consuming enough cruciferous vegetables. The irregular consumption of green and yellow vegetables was found to be significantly higher in 100 men with BPH when compared to 100 men not having BPH, hinting that these vegetables may have beneficial, prophylactic effects.[34]

Laboratory studies have linked Vitamin A deficiency to the development of different kinds of tumors, and have been able to decrease prostate cancer with Vitamin A supplements.[35] The Recommended Daily Allowance of Vitamin A is 5,000 International Units (IU). At the most, do not take more than 10,000 IU a day from all sources (diet plus supplements). An overdose can cause liver damage, lack of appetite, dry skin, hair loss, joint pain, irritability, and headaches.[36] Because the body does not convert beta-carotene to Vitamin A when Vitamin A levels are within normal ranges, eating fruits and vegetables containing beta-carotene will not lead to Vitamin A toxicity.[37]

SAY "YES" TO COOKED TOMATOES

Lycopenes, which are found in tomatoes and give them their red color, act as a strong antioxidant and protection against lung, colon, bladder, pancreas, and prostate tumors, as well as cutting heart attack risk.[38] In order to help reduce an enlarging prostate, the tomatoes must be cooked because lycopene is most easily absorbed when tomatoes or tomato products are cooked, especially in a little oil, according to Dr. Lenore Kohlmeier, professor of epidemiology and nutrition at the School of Public Health and Medicine at the University of North Carolina, Chapel Hill.[39] They also need to be eaten at least five times a week. Could this be why Italian and Greek men have fewer prostate problems than men in other countries? Best sources for cooked tomatoes are tomato sauce, canned tomatoes, tomato paste, and tomato juice.

INCREASE THE GARLIC IN YOUR DIET

Throughout the history of humans, many cultures have used herbs not only for nutrients but also for their health benefits. Garlic *(Allium sativum)* is one of the most medicinal of all the culinary herbs. Its remains have been found in caves used by early man as long as 10,000 years ago. The first garlic prescription was found chiseled in cuneiform on a Sumerian clay tablet dating back to 3000 B.C. The Egyptians used garlic to provide strength and nourishment to the slaves constructing the pyramids.[40]

Garlic's healing qualities have been related to various sulphur compounds it contains (although there are some 75 more), which are the key to its antibiotic and antifungal action (penicillin is also a sulphur compound). Two have received much attention: The first, alliin, has neither smell nor taste nor medicinal effects. So what good is it? Well, when garlic is cut, crushed, or otherwise bruised, alliin makes contact with a catalytic enzyme called allinase, which converts the alliin into allicin, the compound that is not only responsible for garlic's characteristic odor, but many of its potent health benefits. Unfortunately, if left to stand in the air or when cooked, allicin is destroyed.

The sulphur compounds in raw garlic help prevent the liver from generating too much cholesterol, help thin the blood and reduce clotting, inhibit inflammation, protect against the effects of radiation, offer antioxidant protection to cell membranes, and may provide a normalizing effect on the prostate. Garlic and its cousins (onions, scallions, shallots, leeks, and chives) inhibit the production of certain enzymes (lipoxygenase and cyclooxygenase), thus slow-ing the production of prostaglandins, which are involved in the process of inflammation. Many cancers are prostaglandin dependent, which may explain, at least in part, the antitumor properties of the oils of the *allium* family. They also lower cholesterol, triglycerides, and low-density lipoprotein (also known as LDL or "bad" cholesterol) levels while increasing levels of the beneficial high-density lipoprotein or HDL.[41]

Although many nutritionists recommend raw garlic or cooked, uncrushed garlic buds (3 grams, about one clove), at least one herbalist suggests that one gram of dried garlic per day will also be effective.[42]

CONSUME ADEQUATE AMOUNTS OF FIBER

Dietary fiber refers to a wide variety of plant carbohydrates that are not digested by humans. It can be divided into two types: "soluble" (oat bran) fiber and "insoluble" (wheat bran) fiber, with the latter being thought to help reduce the risk for colorectal cancer. Fiber speeds the passage of fecal matter through the intestines, thus reducing the time the body is exposed to toxins. Soluble fiber also helps reduce circulating total cholesterol concentrations.[43]

Researchers in the Department of Internal Medicine at the University of Illinois found that increasing dietary wheat bran by 10 percent (but not 3.3 percent or 6.6 percent) in all forms (hard red, soft white, or finely ground soft white) caused a 65 percent reduction in prostate enlargement.[44]

Good sources of fiber include beans, vegetables, whole grains, and fruits. Rice, another staple in the Asian diet, is an ideal carbohydrate. It has fewer calories and is more filling than bread. Soybean fiber reduces fat levels in the blood; and seaweed contains certain gums that slow fat absorption, as well as providing calcium.

GET ENOUGH VITAMIN D

Some research suggests that by promoting the body's production of Vitamin D, sunlight may protect against prostate cancer. When the incidences of the death of Caucasian men from prostate cancer was examined for 3,073 counties in the United States, the highest mortality rates occurred in those areas with the lowest amount of ultraviolet (UV) radiation (Vitamin D is synthesized in the skin after exposure to sunlight's UV radiation). Deaths from prostate cancer were highest in the Northeast and lowest in the Southwest,[45] while the study we quoted in Chapter 5 showed a broad belt across the entire northern area of the United States as being highest, with the same broad belt across southern United States as being the lowest. This may also explain, in part, the high death rates from prostate cancer death in Scandinavian countries and Canada.[46] The *Johns Hopkins 1997 White Paper on Prostate Disorders* reports a laboratory study that found that concentrations of the active form of Vitamin D change the makeup of prostate cancer cells such that they are less likely to spread.[47]

With the new information we have on the risk of getting skin cancer from being out in the sun, and the fact that as we age, our skin becomes less effective at absorbing vitamin D, health care specialists have been concerned for some time now about the amount of Vitamin D people are getting.

A new study suggests that, in fact, a borderline deficiency of Vitamin D is widespread and not just limited to older adults. Researchers at Massachusetts General Hospital in Boston evaluated the Vitamin D status of 290 people, ages 18 to 98, admitted to the hospital. Fifty-seven percent were deficient in Vitamin D, and 22 percent severely so. When the researchers looked at a subgroup of 77 young and healthy patients under 65 years of age, with no risk factors for Vitamin D deficiency, they found that 42 percent were deficient, and 14 percent severely so.[48]

> The cheapest way to get your daily requirement of Vitamin D is to step outside on a sunny day for 5 to 15 minutes. Most of us accumulate this amount of sunlight as we run errands, go in and out of our workplace, transport our children to their activities, and engage in other daily comings and goings.

In 1997 the recommended Reference Daily Intake (RDI) amount of Vitamin D was doubled to 400 international units (IU) for persons over 50 years of age and tripled to 600 IU for adults over 70. While you might consider a supplement, one of the startling findings of the above study was that 46 percent of those who reported taking a multivitamin were also deficient in Vitamin D. So, even if you take a supplement or a multivitamin, plan to also get more Vitamin D from fish oil, salmon, tuna, sardines, and vitamin D-fortified nonfat milk (although several studies have shown milk to be a shockingly unreliable source of Vitamin D, even when labeled as fortified).[49]

However, if you believe that you must take more Vitamin D, get no more than five times the RDI. Overdose can cause loss of appetite, nausea, weakness, constipation, kidney stones, calcium deposits in the blood vessels, high blood pressure, and kidney failure.[50]

AVOID CAFFEINE, ALCOHOL, AND SPICY FOODS

Most urologists believe that caffeine (a known diuretic), alcohol, and spicy foods can irritate an already enlarged prostate, and suggest that you eliminate them or at least cut back on their use. They can also exacerbate bladder irritation and cause bladder spasms, which, in turn, can cause reflux of urine into the prostatic ducts and contribute to symptoms of nonbacterial prostatitis.[51]

MAKE FRIENDS
WITH THOSE BENEFICIAL ANTIOXIDANTS

Vitamin C (ascorbic acid) is considered by many researchers and nutritionists to be the premier antioxidant, the "number one" vitamin. This essential nutrient has one of the widest ranges of any vitamin of therapeutic applications in the prevention and treatment of disease. High amounts of Vitamin C are found in the prostate gland, and are believed to be important for prostate function.

Vitamin C plays a starring role in preventing much of the damaging effects of free radicals, which are present in tobacco smoke, air pollution, radiation, and herbicides. Excess sun exposure, dietary imbalances, processed foods, and stress also promote damage from free radicals.

Vitamin C, which the body does not manufacture, is destroyed constantly as a result of toxins in foods, pollution, stress, alcohol, and cigarettes. Several *in vitro* (laboratory) studies describe the protective role of Vitamin C against cancer development in general; in the treatment of established cancer, especially estrogen-induced renal cancer,[52] mammary tumors and ultraviolet light-induced skin tumors;[53] and in its effects on prolonging length of survival in terminal cancer. The protective effects of Vitamin C require high doses and long-term treatment.[54] Epidemiological studies wherein the populations ingested much lower doses of Vitamin C (from 60 to 100 mg daily, the FDA-recommended levels) do not show a reduction in the incidence of prostate cancer; however, until recently no studies of any kind had been performed specifically with prostate cancer.[55]

Then, researchers associated with the University of Massachu-

HOW ANTIOXIDANTS WORK AGAINST FREE RADICALS

A normal oxygen atom in the human body contains four pairs of electrons. When oxygen is consumed in the cells, it is typically reduced by four electrons, resulting in water and energy. During the course of normal metabolism, however, a single electron is often lost. The result is a *free radical*, an unstable molecule with a strong drive to replace its missing electron partner. To accomplish this, it will scavenge for an electron from a neighboring molecule, which sets off a chain reaction of cellular deterioration and damage, since the molecule that has had its electron "stolen" becomes a new free radical and also dutifully sets off to attack the nearest cell or molecule to find a partner.

Scientists think it likely that these oxidative reactions are contributing factors in the normal aging process and in a number of degenerative diseases as cells are destroyed and die, or as genes are altered and cells become pathological. Certain vitamins and minerals—especially beta-carotene, Vitamins C and E, selenium, and zinc—act as antioxidants; they are able to give up an electron to the free radical without causing harm to their own molecular structure. In this way they interrupt and ward off some of the short- and long-term harm done by free radicals.

setts Medical Center in Worcester studied the effect of Vitamin C on prostate cancer cells *in vitro,* using cell lines derived from lymph node carcinoma of the prostate and prostatic adenocarcinoma metastasized to brain tissue. They discovered that there is a greater uptake of oxidized Vitamin C by prostate cancer cells and that the Vitamin C "treatment" decreases the number of cancer cells. The higher the Vitamin C concentration, the greater the decrease, which seems to occur through the vitamin's production of hydrogen peroxide, known to damage the cells. The exact means by which this damage occurs is not as yet identified.[56]

Food sources rich in Vitamin C are citrus fruits, strawberries, tomatoes, and red and green peppers. Overdose (more than 10 times the RDI) can cause diarrhea, urinary tract irritation, kidney stones, and bone damage. Vitamin C promotes iron absorption; hence too much C can also cause a toxic accumulation of iron.[57] Excessive iron in the body promotes the formation of free radicals.

Almost as important as Vitamin C in prostate health is *Vitamin E* or *alpha-tocopherol,* one of the most essential vitamins needed by the body. It is a powerful antidote to aging and hardening of tissue through oxidation. It promotes athletic endurance, helps preserve eye health, and is an oxygenator of the heart and all other muscles. It helps to stabilize and protect cell membranes, strengthening them and increasing their resistance to free radicals. A chemoprevention trial investigating lung carcinoma among smokers in Finland serendipitously found a significant reduction in the rate of prostate cancer in 99 men who received Vitamin E, compared to 151 cases who received a placebo.[58]

Many men and women are taking 200–400 International Units (IUs) of d alpha tocopherol (Vitamin E) in order to avoid cardiovascular disorders.[59,60] Good natural sources of Vitamin E are vegetable oils, nuts, whole grains, wheat germ, and asparagus. Overdose can cause headache, nausea, fatigue, giddiness, inflammation of the mouth, chapped lips, gastrointestinal upset, muscle weakness, low blood sugar, and blurred vision.[61]

GATHER IN THE GINKGO

Having appeared about 200 million years ago, the ginkgo *(Ginkgo biloba)* is the oldest living species of tree on earth, and contains "ginkgolides," a kind of bioflavonoid that has a unique chemical structure with proven antioxidant and vasodilating properties. Not found in any other growing thing, ginkgolides decrease blood stickiness and increase the elasticity of tiny blood vessels. Although no studies have been done establishing the effect of ginkgo on prostate health, it does have potent antioxidant properties that block free radical damage to cells and may, therefore, assist in protecting the prostate.

TO ZINC OR NOT TO ZINC?

Zinc is a trace mineral that occurs naturally throughout the earth in plants and animals and, therefore, in the foods we eat. It is essential to life, since every cell in the body requires zinc to multiply. Zinc stimulates mental activity, regulates appetite, and improves muscle strength and endurance. Because it is also a natural sunscreen, zinc preparations are often used to protect lips and skin from the sun's rays.

Overall, zinc increases T-lymphocyte production and enhances other white blood cell functions necessary for a healthy immune system and for regulating the body's response to injury and infection. Serum (blood) levels of zinc were shown to be significantly lower in 19 patients with prostate cancer, compared to 27 men with BPH.[62] Some researchers have found that not only is zinc effective against certain types of bacteria, but that patients with chronic prostatitis have little or no zinc in their prostatic secretions.[63] Experts differ as to whether the drop in zinc concentration precedes bacterial invasion, or the bacteria cause a drop in the amount.

Although zinc is actually found in the body in only small amounts (2 to 2.5 grams), according to Melvyn Werbach, M.D., author of *Healing with Food,* the level of zinc in a man's prostate is higher than in any other organ of his body, possibly because it is required for the metabolism of the male hormones within the prostate. The prostate uses 10 times more zinc than any other organ in a man's body. An enlarged prostate causes a decrease in the binding of zinc to the cells of the prostate.[64] Stress, burns, surgery, and weight loss will all increase bodily losses of zinc, and alcohol use increases urinary losses of zinc.

Even though prostatic zinc levels may be elevated and blood zinc levels may be normal, the prostatic cells may actually be zinc-deprived, says Dr. Werbach. At least two preliminary studies done in the 1970s showed that zinc supplementation reduced the size of the prostate, but none have been done on humans since.[65]

In 1993 a team of researchers showed that the prostate weight and 5-alpha-reductase activity of sexually mature rats was reduced when neutralized zinc (zinc gluconate plus arginine) was injected directly into the prostate.[66] A 1976 study indicated that the values of zinc in normal tissue BPH of human prostates were similar while zinc concentrations were significantly lower in neoplastic (tumorous) tissue.[67] When serum zinc and Vitamin A levels were measured in 27 patients with BPH and 19 patients with prostate cancer, a significantly lower level of serum zinc was found in the cancer group than the BPH group. There was, however, so much overlap between the values of the two groups that the zinc level on its own could not be considered helpful as a predictor of carcinoma of the prostate.[68]

Authorities who suggest zinc as a supplement seem to vary in their understanding of the function of zinc. One believes that it reduces the levels of prolactin, "the hormone that encourages the prostate to swell."[69] Prolactin is produced in the pituitary, and zinc certainly has been shown to inhibit prolactin secretion in the pituitary of female rats.[70]

Other researchers believe that zinc regulates the metabolism of the 5-alpha-reduction of testosterone in the prostate. Low levels of zinc increase 5-alpha-reductase activity, while higher concentrations inhibit its metabolism (as does the drug finasteride).[71]

Zinc can be found naturally in oysters (more than 10 times the amount of other sources), lamb chops, lean red meats, and soybeans.

Fish and poultry contain fair levels, although the zinc content in foods can be depleted by cooking. Whole grains constitute another important source of zinc, especially wheat germ, whole wheat, rye, and oats that have not been processed, inasmuch as the zinc is found mainly in the germ and bran coverings. Beans, cheese, and nuts—pecans, Brazil nuts, and especially unsalted, raw pumpkin seeds—are fairly good sources, as are ginger, mustard, chili powder, and black pepper.

Researchers and nutritionists are engaged in an ongoing debate, however, about the kind and quantity of *supplemental* zinc to take. Some urologists recommend zinc sulfate tablets, saying that zinc glutamate, which many people take to fight colds, is not effective. Others warn that taking extremely large amounts of zinc may make it more difficult for the body to defend itself against infection and cancer.[72]

A diet high in iron and folic acid reduces the body's ability to absorb zinc, while picolinic acid and *dietary* Vitamin B-6 (found in liver, poultry, fish, egg yolks, bananas, and potatoes) increase zinc absorption, at least in rats.[73] Zinc also needs to be balanced by extra Vitamin A, which can be obtained by diet or from a beta-carotene supplement.[74]

Because zinc can interfere with copper absorption, anyone taking zinc supplements needs to balance their diet with supplemental copper. The copper should not be taken at the same time as the zinc, however, and not too much should be consumed, because high amounts of copper in water, food, or supplements will also reduce zinc levels. The suggested zinc-to-copper ratio is about 15 to 1.[75]

HEED POSSIBLE HERBAL/MEDICATION INTERACTIONS

Although herbal preparations are frequently prescribed in European countries, you should not use them without first determining from your doctor whether their use will interact or interfere with any other prescription or over-the-counter medications you are taking. Also advise your doctor about any supplements you take.

Many herbs, including ginkgo, garlic, ginger, ginseng, and white willow bark, are blood-thinners. If you combine them with prescription anticoagulant drugs, or aspirin, they could cause bleeding or even stroke, according to Dr. Varro Tyler, distinguished professor emeritus of pharmacognosy at Purdue University in West Lafayette, Indiana.[76] If your doctor can't tell you whether specific herbs could cause such effects, consult a trained herbalist.

KEEP YOUR CHOLESTEROL LEVEL IN CHECK

Throughout this chapter we mention various dietary factors that influence serum levels of cholesterol. We do that because DHT and testosterone more easily bind to prostate receptors when cholesterol is high in the prostate.

Cholesterol, a waxy, fatty substance manufactured in the liver and found in all animal tissue, comes from foods derived from animal sources; that is, meat, dairy products, eggs (especially the yolks, one of which can contain as much as 213 mg of cholesterol), and fats. You need some cholesterol, but your body can manufacture most of the cholesterol it needs to build cell membranes, create insulating sheaths around nerve fibers, and to serve as a basis for the production of certain hormones.

Cholesterol is carried in the body by two forms of proteins: low-density lipoproteins (LDL), and high-density lipoproteins (HDL). Unfortunately, LDL is one of the major causes of plaque buildup in blood vessels. Too much LDL cholesterol in the blood causes plaque to be deposited on artery walls, greatly narrowing them and increasing blood pressure and contributing to heart disease.[77]

AVOID DECONGESTANTS AND ANTIHISTAMINES

Learn to read the fine print. The most popular decongestants and antihistamines (e.g., Actifed, Benadryl) all carry warnings not to use them if a person has an enlarged prostate of BPH. They are notorious for provoking the prostate, causing it to contract, which, of course, decreases urine flow. This is why for persons who need to use decongestants and antihistamines, Cernitin to reduce the prostate size is an important choice.

Some antidepressants, such as Elavil or Norpramin, digestive tract drugs (Donnatal), narcotic analgesics, anticonvulsants, or Parkinson's disease medications may also cause difficulties. Before you take any over-the-counter drugs—or for that matter, any prescribed medications—check with your doctor or pharmacist if you are not sure what their effect is on the prostate.[78]

DON'T SMOKE

There is some evidence that cigarette smoking may indirectly affect the size of the enlarging prostate. The association between cigarette smoking and prostatic volume was investigated in 68 men with BPH by assessing changes in serum levels of four specific androgens. One of the androgens—oestradiol—showed significantly higher levels for smokers than nonsmokers.[79]

Cigarette smoke is high in cadmium, a toxic heavy metal, which is markedly higher in the cancerous prostate. There have also been reports, largely anecdotal, of a positive association between smoking and prostate cancer. However, a study of 1,097 prostate cancer cases and 3,250 matched controls admitted between 1969 and 1991 to U.S. hospitals, found no association between prostate cancer and former or current smoking, age started smoking, number of years of smoking, cigarettes per day smoked, number of years since quitting, and lifetime tar exposure.[80] This is *not* to say that smoking is not related to other types of cancers.

• • •

You've seen in this chapter that what you put into your body can actually strengthen (or weaken) your immune system, and can help fortify you against getting prostate cancer, as well as heart disease, stroke, and other major killer diseases. Your body needs many nutrients to continue functioning in top form.

As we said at the beginning of this chapter, a diet designed to promote prostate health and prevent prostate cancer is also a healthy diet. It entails a variety of foods—especially those that contain antioxidants—and requires you to keep your weight under control.

Any kind of change, especially one that involves your daily eating habits, can feel stressful and uncomfortable at first. So, as you choose more foods high in nutrients (such as vegetables, grains, and fresh fruit), think of this new regimen as strengthening your immune system. Some determination and self-control may be required, but your immune system will love you for it.

To provide interested readers with the latest information about a wide range of health topics—including the effects of diet and BPH—Brenda Adderly, the coauthor of this book, publishes a monthly newsletter entitled *Health Watch*. Contents include healthy recipes, nutritional information, and research updates about many health-related issues. See the back page for more details.

7

PROSTATE CANCER

Is there really a prostate cancer epidemic?

*

Why are we hearing more about prostate cancer now?

*

What causes prostate cancer?

*

What influences the development of prostate cancer?

*

Why would a man need a prostate-specific antigen (PSA) test?

*

What are the treatments for prostate cancer?

*

What is a radical prostatectomy?

I t may seem odd to devote a chapter to prostate cancer in a book about BPH—and especially so when we clearly stated in Chapter 1 that BPH does not necessarily lead to prostate cancer. To be perfectly clear, let us reiterate: *BPH is not prostate cancer, and having an enlarged prostate does not mean that a man is more likely to get prostate cancer.* However, many people are still confused about the differences between the two conditions, and some people unwittingly refer to them interchangeably.

So as not to scare people unnecessarily, we will briefly discuss the latest developments, warning signs, and treatment options in prostate cancer. Also, in the interests of comprehensiveness for a book called *The Prostate Cure,* we want to include as much information as possible on this problematic organ.

Let's start with a question. What do former senator Bob Dole, actor Sidney Poitier, singers Robert Goulet and Harry Belafonte, and retired general Norman Schwarzkopf have in common? If you guessed from the title of this chapter that all five have been diagnosed as having prostate cancer, you're 100 percent correct. *Time* magazine called it "The Man's Cancer" that "strikes at the very core of masculinity."

The statistics regarding prostate cancer are almost overwhelming and certainly not to be ignored. In 1985, 85,000 cases of prostate cancer were recorded. By 1988, the annual number had risen to 99,000. During the past decade prostate cancer numbers have continued to rise—one doctor has called the growing incidence an "epidemic"—and the prediction is that one in five American men will develop prostate cancer. The American Cancer Society estimates that more than 317,000 new cases of prostate cancer were discovered in 1996[1]—an increase of more than 300 percent in less than 10 years—with 370,000 new cases projected for 1997.[2] A new case of prostate cancer is diagnosed every two minutes, and an associated death occurs every 15 minutes.[3] According to Dr. Curtis Mettlin of the Roswell Park Cancer Institute in Buffalo, New York, these figures represent "the most dramatic change in cancer incidence to occur in this century."[4]

These rising figures are actually not due to a real epidemic, but occur in part because men are living longer, giving them a higher chance of developing prostate cancer. More influential in the dramatic upsurge in discovery of prostate cancer is the development of modern detection technology and, in particular, the use of a new

> *Current rapid increases in the success of diagnoses are having the effect of leaving experts arguing—and patients confused—about how and when to treat prostate cancer.*

blood test. Called the prostate-specific antigen (PSA) test, it makes diagnosis easier and earlier—there are usually no symptoms of prostate cancer in its early stages—often long before the tumor becomes palpable with a digital rectal exam (DRE). (At least one doctor has estimated that by the time a solid tumor is either measurable, palpable, or visible, the cancer cell population is at least one billion, and a 99 percent success rate in eradicating the tumor still leaves behind 10 million viable cancer cells.)[5]

Regardless of the reasons, and whether you call it an epidemic or the result of modern detection technology, the changes occurring now and in the next few years are of such tremendous magnitude that they will have important consequences for patterns of prostate diagnoses and patient care.[6]

In contrast to breast cancer, which doubles its size every three months, half of all prostate cancers take more than five years to double their size.[7] While it is the most common type of cancer in men, prostate cancer is, at the same time, the slowest-growing common cancer in humans.

Some doctors fear that if prostate cancer is found as a result of an elevated PSA, many men who might live out the course of their life without ever knowing they have cancer will, at the least, live with a higher level of anxiety and, more significantly, may be urged into unnecessary and painful treatments or surgery that may actually shorten their lives or reduce their quality of life. Others believe that an early PSA may be used to alert a man that lifestyle changes and a new level of vigilance are necessary.

It is often said, though not quite true, that most men with prostate cancer die with, rather than of, the disease—because it is possible to die of other disorders before prostate cancer becomes life-threatening. The statement is misleading, however, and may offer false hope to some men, because it *is* a fact that men can and *do* die of prostate cancer. In fact, prostate cancer is the most common cause of cancer death in males over the age of 50 years. One out of 11 men in the United States will die of prostate cancer. That means that of the estimated 10 million men now between 50 and 75 years of age, prostate cancer will probably kill almost one million.[8] Many well-known personalities have died of it already. These include actors Telly Savalas, Bill Bixby, Dick Sargent, and Don Ameche. Tennis player Bobby Riggs lost his battle with prostate cancer, as did François Mitterrand, former president of France.[9]

POSSIBLE CAUSAL FACTORS OF PROSTATE CANCER

No one yet knows exactly what causes prostate cancer. As with all cancers, the first step is some sequence of events that produces an alteration or mutation in the genetic makeup of a cell.[10] Then something has to occur that stimulates the growth of the abnormal cell.

> *One possible key factor in the development of prostate cancer may be the absence of tumor-suppressing genes, due to genetic factors that cause them to mutate or to be obliterated.*[11]

Various speculations as to that unknown but influential "something" that causes a cancer cell to begin to grow include an imbalance of male sex hormones or the presence of a virus.[12]

Age, family history, and race are all important risk factors in prostate cancer, and it's beginning to appear that diet and exposure to sunlight may play some slight role as well, although the data are still inconclusive.

The incidence of prostate cancer increases with age. In this country, autopsy studies show that 40 percent of men older than 50 years and 70 percent of men in their 80s harbor prostate cancer. This means that there are more than eight million undetected cases of prostate cancer at any one time.[13]

About 10 percent of prostate cancer is inherited.[14] The risk grows with the number of affected relatives, or when cancer is discovered in another family member before the age of 55.[15] If a man's father had prostate cancer, for instance, he's at twice the risk. If his brother *also* developed it, the risk rises to five times greater—and goes up depending on the number of affected relatives and the age at which they develop cancer.[16] For men from families with a history of prostate cancer, the chances of developing it may be as high as 50 percent. Several lines of evidence, including determination of specific genes and examination of family lifestyle of susceptible families, suggest the likelihood that "familial prostate cancer" is due to an inherited susceptibility—a "high-risk" gene, if you will—rather than to family lifestyle.[17] Interestingly, prostate cancer can be inherited from the men in either the father's or the mother's family.[18]

African-American men living in the United States have a 37 percent higher risk of contracting prostate cancer than do Caucasian men, and a higher rate of prostate-cancer-related death as well.[19] National data show that the lifetime risk of developing prostate cancer is 1 in 9 in African-Americans, and 1 in 11 for Caucasians.[20] Like their Asian counterparts remaining in Japan, black men living in Africa have a lower risk of developing prostate cancer. Once both groups emigrate, their risk of developing prostate cancer increases considerably, causing some to attribute a causal relationship between the cancer and the high-fat diet consumed by Americans.[21]

Some researchers have attributed the higher incidence of prostate cancer in blacks to delays in detection and treatment; however, in populations with equal access to medical care, such as military personnel, studies still have found higher proportions of prostate cancer and poorer survival rates among blacks than among whites. Speculation is that black men are not only at higher risk of prostate cancer than white men, but they are also at higher risk for the more aggressive forms of the disease, and that this risk is likely to be genetically determined.[22]

The development of prostate cancer can be linked to the sexual hormones, but again, it is not clear if this is influenced by the genetics of race or by diet. The testosterone levels in young black men are about 15 percent higher than those in young white men (but when black American men eat a vegetarian diet, their hormonal levels decrease).[23] Likewise, Dutch men have higher levels of testosterone than do Japanese men. American men have higher levels of dihydrotestosterone (DHT) metabolites than Japanese men, but it is not

A study conducted at Harvard University showed that dietary fat may determine in part whether or not prostate tumors remain tiny and nontroublesome or progress to a life-threatening stage. Men with a high fat intake had a 79 percent increased risk of advanced cancer compared to men with the lowest level of fat intake.[24]

> *When several studies in the early 1990s suggested that having a vasectomy increased the risk of prostate cancer, the National Institutes of Health convened a blue-ribbon panel to investigate. After reviewing the data, including papers presented at meetings of the American Urological Association, the panel concluded that vasectomies and prostate cancer are not causally linked.[25] Also, no association has been found between prostate cancer and the presence of BPH.*

clear whether this is due to the fact that Japanese men have smaller prostates, which contribute less DHT to the blood.[26] Beyond these figures, prostate cancer indiscriminately crosses socioeconomic, educational, and occupational lines, but perhaps not locale. One study showed a north-south differential, with the heaviest areas of prostate cancer extending in a broad belt across the northern United States and the lightest across the southern states.[27]

THE PROSTATE-SPECIFIC ANTIGEN (PSA) TEST

Like BPH, prostate cancer is a silent disease. Men may never exhibit some of the typical symptoms of cancer that would cause them to seek a doctor's opinion: pain in the bones, weight loss, chronic fatigue, or even problems with urination. Fortunately, they now don't have to wait for the appearance of painful symptoms.

First developed in the 1980s to determine whether treatment of cancer had removed all malignant tissue, the prostate-specific antigen (PSA) test was approved by the FDA in 1994 to screen for the presence of cancer. It measures the level in the blood of an enzyme produced exclusively by prostate cells. This prostate-specific antigen is secreted during ejaculation, and one of its functions is to liquefy semen so that sperm are released.

THE CANCER SCREENING DILEMMA

At what age cancer screening should begin is a very controversial issue among physicians. According to research findings by the American College of Physicians (ACP), prostate cancer screening is not for everyone. The group reached this conclusion following an intense literature examination and analysis, and their three-part study was published in the March 1997 issue of the *Annals of Internal Medicine*.[31] It is a controversial finding, however, and at least one doctor argues that the ACP's analysis of benefits and risks of screening were not reliable or even very useful. He states that their review of only certain studies from the literature limited their findings, and that the significance of complications was not accurately represented.[32]

In the late 1920s Dr. H. H. Young first recognized that the digital rectal exam (DRE) was a principal means of diagnosing cancer at the time. Most doctors recommend that starting at 40 years of age, men should have a DRE as part of their annual checkup.

With the advent of PSA testing, some doctors believe that almost all malignant cancers of the prostate can be detected if both DRE and PSA are used together in initial screening. Hence, most doctors recommended that all men between the ages of 50 and 75 years who have no disease that would reduce their actuarial survival to less than 12 years should have both an annual digital rectal examination and serum PSA testing. Most doctors continue to recommend an annual screening for men younger than 50 years of age who carry a risk factor for prostate cancer.

While the PSA test is the best marker to date for indicating the existence of cancer, about two-thirds of its positive results turn out to be false alarms,[28] especially in the 2.5 to 10.0 ng/ml (nanograms, or billionths of a gram, per milliliter of blood) range.[29] In addition, large amounts of BPH tissue or its rapid growth can cause such an elevation of serum PSA that it may mask the rise caused by cancer. Still PSA testing is being touted as playing a major role in decreasing the death rate from prostate cancer because of early detection.

As the prostate enlarges with age, the growing number of cells results in a steady but slight rise in PSA count. Very little PSA continues to enter the blood, however, unless some abnormality of the prostate creates a means for the enzyme to pass into the blood stream. Normally PSA is secreted and disposed of through tiny ducts in the prostate that drain into the urethra, but with prostate cancer, the ductal system doesn't drain into the urethra. According to the well-known urologist Dr. Patrick C. Walsh, affiliated with Johns Hopkins, the PSA builds up, leaks out of the prostate, and shows up in the bloodstream.[30]

WHY A RISE IN PSA CAN SUGGEST THE POSSIBILITY OF CANCER

Just three years after his triumph in the Gulf War, General H. Norman Schwarzkopf visited his urologist, because "I felt something not quite right." His doctor performed a routine rectal exam and a PSA test, and felt confident that he could detect any cancer with these tests. Although Schwarzkopf's PSA level was "below the radar," the doctor performed an ultrasound and a biopsy to finally reach his diagnosis: prostate cancer.

For PSA tests, a reading of 4 is close to a "magic" number, because it is commonly used as a cutoff level. In general, PSA readings below 4 ng/ml indicate that cancer is highly unlikely (Schwarz-kopf's count was 1.8 ng/m).[33] This is because PSA is prostate-specific, not cancer-specific; hence, like General Schwarzkopf, you can have prostate cancer and still have a low PSA level.[34] Two doctors from the University of Oklahoma Health Sciences Center estimate that about 16 percent of men with prostate cancer will both have PSA values falling within the range of normal PSA and a normal digital rectal exam.[35]

When the PSA count rises to or above 4 ng/ml, the probability of some sort of prostate trouble, especially cancer, rises threefold for intracapsular tumors (within the prostate capsule) and as much as fivefold for extracapsular (outside the capsule) tumors.[36] Apparently, gram-for-gram the average prostate cancer produces at least 10 times the amount of PSA as normal prostatic tissue,[37] although both BPH and prostatitis can elevate PSA levels somewhat, leaving the 4 to 10 ng/ml range to be defined by some urologists as "the gray zone."[38] In fact, about 38 to 40 percent of patients with a PSA level less than 4 ng/ml have a localized prostate cancer,[39] and about 30 percent of men with PSA levels between 4 to 10 ng/ml have cancers that have already extended through the prostatic capsule or metastasized at the time of diagnosis.[40]

With each subsequent increase in the PSA count beyond 4 ng/ml—or a sudden, dramatic jump in the count—the likelihood of cancer likewise steadily increases, and then soars when the count goes above 20. For instance, the chance of prostatic cancer is 20 to 50 percent in those with PSA levels between 4 to 10 ng/ml. Above 10 ng/ml, the odds rise to between 50 and 75 percent, and with a PSA count exceeding 20, the probability rises to 90 percent. Once the diagnosis of a prostatic cancer is made and the patient is treated, the PSA then becomes a very sensitive marker for identifying tumor recurrence and/or metastasis.[41]

WHAT "FREE" PSA VALUES ARE
AND WHAT THEY REVEAL

Doctors are constantly working to make the PSA test a more specific diagnostic test. One promising area of research lies in defining, or distinguishing between, the amount of "bound" versus "unbound" or free molecules of PSA. PSA, which is produced only in the epithelial cells of the prostate,[42] actively attacks other proteins yet is somewhat restrained by inhibitors in the bloodstream that prevent it from breaking down proteins. In other words it is "bound." Researchers began to suspect that the amount of bound PSA may be higher in men with prostate cancer, whereas those with BPH have more of the free form.[43] Numerous studies showed that a diagnosis of prostate cancer occurred in approximately one out of three men who had an ultrasound-guided biopsy following a PSA level of greater than 4.0 ng/ml.[44]

Gradually research began to accrue that has now confirmed that determining the percent of free PSA and the proportion of free-PSA-to-total-PSA enhances the ability of PSA testing to distinguish between prostate cancer and BPH. Men with prostate cancer have a lower percentage of free PSA than men with BPH.[45]

In one French study, comparing the serum samples of 31 histologically (by microscope) confirmed prostate cancers with 74 histo-

> *Doctors from Mayo Clinic have heralded the comparison of the proportion of free-to-total PSA as a "new era" in the detection of prostate cancer. It may contribute to a reduction in unnecessary invasive techniques[46] by as much as 30 percent.[47]*

logically confirmed untreated BPH, both total PSA and the proportion of free-to-total PSA significantly differentiated between patients with prostate cancer and patients with BPH. In men with total PSA values between 4.0 and 10.0 ng/ml, the ratio of free-to-total PSA significantly differentiated between those men with benign and those with malignant conditions, even where the rectal digital examination was normal.[48]

Researchers in Barcelona, Spain, measured the free and total PSA concentrations in the blood of 156 patients with BPH and 74 patients with prostate cancer. Patients with prostate cancer had a significantly lower free-to-total PSA ratio than patients with BPH. The authors conclude that in patients with a total PSA level between 4 mg and 25 mg, the free-to-total PSA ratio demonstrated better diagnostic utility than total PSA alone.[49] Still, the medical community awaits an international standardization, not only for the sum of free PSA but also for the free-to-total PSA ratio.[50]

As it stands now, the literature indicates that the percent of free PSA has the greatest clinical significance in persons whose total PSA values range from 1.5 to 10.0. When the total PSA value is in the normal range, between 2.5 to 4.0 ng/ml, the percentage value of free PSA increases the likelihood of cancer detection. When the total PSA level ranges between 4.1 to 10.0, the percent of free PSA makes PSA a more specific test; that is, it eliminates the need for unnecessary prostate biopsies.[51]

In an attempt to further understand the components of the free-to-total PSA, researchers at Stanford University have discovered a number of differences between the PSA from seminal fluid and that from BPH nodules. They suggest that antibodies produced against PSA in BPH tissue will likely be useful in discriminating prostate cancer from BPH.[52]

Two additional approaches for using PSA levels to distinguish prostate cancer from BPH have to do with the amount and rate of change in PSA. The first is that *as a man ages, his prostate gets larger;* therefore PSA rates differentiated as to age (age-related PSA values) should make the PSA a more selective marker for tumor and reduce the number of unnecessary diagnostic procedures. Several urologists have defined the *upper limits* of age-specific reference range as 0.0–2.5 ng/ml for men in their 50s, 0.0–3.5 ng/ml for men in their 60s, 0.0–4.5 ng/ml for men in their 70s, and 0.0–6.5 for men in their 80s. These ranges are suggested provided a man has either a normal digital rectal exam or ultrasound, or in the face of an abnormality, that he has a negative ultrasound-guided biopsy.[53] One urologist argues, however, that the recommended age-specific reference ranges are limited because they delay the detection of curable cancers in men age 60 to 73 who may be legitimate candidates for curative surgery.[54] And, indeed, one study showed that a PSA greater than 4.0 ng/ml detected markedly more prostate cancer cases than age-specific PSA.[55]

The second approach, that of examining the rate of change from year to year, is based on the assumption that a man's *yearly rate of PSA change* will be much greater if he has prostate cancer than if he has BPH.

Controversy continues over the effectiveness of the PSA test due to the number of both "false negative" and "false positive" results. With a "false negative" result, the PSA number will show "normal" even when cancer is actually present. "False positive" results occur when there are high levels of PSA present with no cancer. One of the reasons for a false positive result can be the growth of benign prostatic tissue (BPH), as we saw in Chapter 1. Other reasons include a temporary rise in PSA due to prostatitis or a urinary tract infection, and a major trauma or injury to the prostate (surgery or biopsy). Subsequent biopsies to check for cancer can be uncomfortable and expensive.

AFTER A HIGH PSA, WHAT'S NEXT?

Typically, as with General Schwarzkopf, if cancer is suspected or an elevated PSA is discovered, the next steps in evaluation and diagnosis consist of viewing the prostate with a transrectal ultrasound (TRUS), and taking tissue samples (needle biopsies) from several of its regions for microscopic diagnosis. During a transrectal ultrasound, a probe inserted in the rectum sends out sound waves that bounce off the prostate. Via computer they create a picture called a sonogram, where most prostate cancers appear less dense than surrounding tissue.[56] Approximately 50 percent of biopsied prostate nodules are found to be malignant.[57]

In addition to finding small cancers that may not be found otherwise, a major advantage of transrectal ultrasound is that it allows a doctor to more accurately direct biopsy needles to the right bit of tissue to be tested and, thanks to technology, to use smaller, less painful needles to capture the core of abnormal-looking tissue rather than just a few cells. Prior to ultrasound's development, urologists could not see what they were doing and had to guess whether they were getting the right tissue.

Diagnosing prostate cancer at an early stage is often difficult,

Although a high PSA or an abnormal digital rectal exam may be the major reason for prescribing a transrectal ultrasound, the procedure is also able to detect cancers that can't be felt with the rectal exam and are still confined to the prostate. It is, however, neither quick nor cheap and is only as good as the skill of the doctor using it.

since a solid mass has yet to form. The cancer cells are spread diffusely through the prostate, so the cancer can easily be missed with a digital rectal exam (DRE)—formerly the only, and relatively inadequate, way to determine if a man had prostate cancer. Too often, by the time a doctor can feel changes in the prostate with a DRE, the cancer has progressed too far for effective treatment. Further, it has been estimated that when the DRE alone is used for cancer detection, 30 to 40 percent of cancers are missed.[59]

The addition of these two screening procedures (PSA test and transrectal ultrasound) has made a great deal of difference in the reliability of catching prostate cancer before it has metastasized (spread to other locations). Although doctors are increasingly ordering ultrasounds and biopsies for men whose PSAs are between 4 and 10 ng/ml, some consider this as overreacting.

ALL PROSTATE CANCERS GET A "GRADE"

Dr. Marc Garnick, a Harvard Medical School professor and leading cancer specialist, says that cancer cells have two unique qualities. First, when compared to other cells in the body, which typically last only a few weeks and then are replaced by new cells, cancer cells have the capacity to multiply indefinitely. They are, he writes, "quite simply . . . a collection of abnormal cells that have forgotten how to die."[60] Making cancer cells even more dangerous is a second unique quality—they can detach themselves from their original site and travel to other parts of the body. This is what doctors mean when they say a cancer has "metastasized."

When prostate cancer spreads, it is more likely to enter the bones than the lungs and liver, common metastatic sites for other cancers. It becomes a particularly devastating and painful disease, with severe pain, especially in the lower back, hips, and upper parts of the thighs. If the cancer spreads to the spine, it may cause compression of the spinal cord, resulting in such symptoms as numbness of the legs, muscular weakness, difficulty in walking, and in severe cases, inability to walk or move the legs (paralysis).[61]

When prostate cancer is discovered, it is "graded" or classified depending on what it looks like and how it behaves, and that may require more tests before a final determination can be reached. Some of these tests could include a bone scan, a computerized axial tomography (CAT) scan, and magnetic resonance imaging to determine if the cancer has spread outside the prostate into lymph nodes or bones.

The classification system that assigns cancers a "grade" or number that predicts prognosis and outcome is called the Gleason scoring system or grading scale. Tumors are assigned a grade from 1 to 5 on the basis of abnormalities in the prostate glands, on the differentiation of cancer cells, and on how clearly the tumor margin is defined. Prostatic cancer can be identified by cell type. Tumor cells showing some characteristics of a cell type are classified as moderately differentiated, and those with little or no characteristics of a cell type are classified as poorly differentiated.[62]

The sum of the two most dominant patterns, plus the secondary pattern of the three provides the total Gleason score (a range of 2 to 10). A Gleason score from 2 to 4 correlates with a well-differentiated cancer; a score of 5 to 6 reflects a moderately differentiated cancer; and a score of 7 to 10 represents a poorly differentiated cancer. The poorer the differentiation of cancer cells, the worse the prognosis.[63]

Another blood test, the man's PAP, may be used to determine the amount of prostatic acid phosphatase (hence PAP) circulating in the blood. PAP levels are generally elevated in men with spreading prostate cancer, although, once again, BPH, prostatitis, hepatitis, pneumonia, and certain cholesterol-lowering drugs can also raise them.[64] A second disadvantage of PAP is that it is not specific to the prostate; other organs can produce it. For these reasons, many urologists have virtually abandoned the use of PAP in favor of PSA testing.[65] Statistics collected by the Commission on Cancer of the American College of Surgeons shows that use of the PAP as a laboratory measure obtained at the time of diagnosis decreased from 62.4 percent of patients in 1984 to 47.0 percent in 1990.[66]

A LIFESAVING THOUGH FORBIDDING SURGERY

The choice of treatment for prostate cancer depends on the extent of the disease, as well as the age and general health of the person. Often the initial decision regarding treatment will be based on weighing the life expectancy against the possibility of death from prostate cancer.

Every form of treatment currently available has significant risks and possible side effects. If the cancer has remained contained in the prostate, then typically it is regarded as curable, although the "cures" may seem agonizingly drastic to some: surgery (removal of the prostate) and/or radiation therapy. Unfortunately, too, the surgery holds the potential for leaving a man incontinent or impotent. Some 40 percent of patients will be impotent from the time of their operation.[67] Doctors argue that these conditions are simply less important than the loss of life. As Dr. Patrick C. Walsh writes, "Potency assumes a lower rung on the ladder of priorities in the face of a life-threatening disease."[68]

Given that position, doctors can advise that urine control usually returns, and, that the risk of severe incontinence is between 2 to 5 percent, while the chance of continuing mild incontinency is between 20 to 50 percent. This means that for about half the men who have prostate surgery, pads or adult diapers will become "essential wardrobe items."[69]

> *The good news is that starting in 1995 a whole host of medications began to be developed that didn't require injections or implantations to restore potency. Clinical trials are underway, and some are already under FDA review. By the time this book is published, there may be even more.*[70]

Men are equally as cavalierly advised that the surgery's resulting impotency, which reporter Leon Jaroff calls "an even more intimate threat to a man's life,"[71] can be taken care of in one of three ways: using a device that temporarily creates a vacuum around the penis, self-injections of drugs into the penis to assist in erection, or implantation of a prosthetic device within the penis. All three are "safe" doctors say, but the very casualness of the statement often belies the fact that men find, once they have made a choice and undertaken surgery, that those options aren't as successful as was implied. "Some of the things that we read about don't return as quickly as advertised," Bob Dole is quoted as saying in a sidebar to a *Time* magazine cover story.[72]

TREATMENTS FOR PROSTATE CANCER: WATCHFUL WAITING

When prostate cancer is discovered in a very early stage, or a man is elderly and the cancer not likely to spread during his lifetime, then "watchful waiting" may be indicated, with specific cancer treatment undertaken only when problems arise. This option, also called "active surveillance," is particularly desirable in situations where treatment might be more risky than the disease; that is, when there is an absence of symptoms and/or the presence of other more threatening medical situations.

Doctors differ considerably in their approval of this "nontreatment." Naturally the more surgery-prone physicians lean in the direction of early removal of the prostate, while the more conservative ones tell us that for any man whose life expectancy is less than 10 years, the surgery may offer only unnecessary discomfort and incapacity.

Oncologists point out that as many as 4 out of 10 men who reach the age of 50 have at least some cancerous cells in their prostate, which will result in higher PSA readings, yet only 8 percent will eventually develop symptoms that affect their quality of life, and only 3 percent will die of the cancer.[73]

Some prostate cancers have a creepingly slow growth rate. Half of all prostate cancers take more than five years to double their size.[74] In addition, autopsies of men who have died from causes other than prostate cancer show that 70 percent of men over 80 have nontroublesome prostate cancers.[75]

RADICAL PROSTATECTOMY

The only potentially promising cure as long as the cancer is still localized within the prostate is the radical prostatectomy, and it certainly has drawbacks of its own. The long-term statistics are not in, so there is no proof as yet that radical prostatectomy saves lives, although many men opt for the risk of surgery to the risk of doing nothing.[76] The results of total prostatectomy so far published suggest that the disease will not be controlled in at least 20 percent of patients.[77]

Whether you and your doctor choose a radical prostatectomy depends in part on your age and where you live. Statistics kept by the American College of Surgeons' Commission on Cancer indicate that patients younger than 55 were approximately seven times more likely to receive radical prostatectomy, compared to patients in the 75 to 79 age range.[78] In part this is due to a common recommendation that because of the natural course of prostate cancer, radical prostatectomy should be limited to otherwise healthy men with a life expectancy of more than 10 years.[79] The data also show that in 1990 the highest proportion of localized prostate cancer patients treated by radical prostatectomy (35.4 percent) were from the Pacific region. The lowest use of this procedure was reported from hospitals in the New England (21.5 percent) and Mid-Atlantic (20.1 percent) regions.[80]

The never-popular surgery, developed at the turn-of-the century at Johns Hopkins Hospital in Baltimore, Maryland, was refined considerably in the 1980s, also by Johns Hopkins surgeon Dr. Patrick Walsh. Not all urology surgeons are skilled or experienced in the newer techniques, although the numbers are steadily increasing.

Until Dr. Walsh's pioneering approach, the two nerve bundles controlling erection—which lie on either side of the prostate—were invariably destroyed during a prostatectomy, rendering a man impotent. Dr. Walsh's "nerve-sparing" technique requires that they be detached from the gland before its removal, and left intact unless the cancer has spread to them. Journalist Leon Jaroff writes that Dr. Walsh reports that as many as 90 percent of men under 50 will regain potency.[81]

Whether or not the nerves that stimulate erections can be saved, impotence will be a factor in a man's life for anywhere from six to 18 months following surgery, and even if the nerves are spared, doctors other than Dr. Walsh estimate the success rate for future erections to be somewhere between 40 to 72 percent. (These rates are higher when the patients rather than their surgeons assessed their sexual function.) A questionnaire study of 739 Medicare patients revealed impotence rates of 89 percent.[82]

Make no mistake. A radical prostatectomy is major surgery (the operation lasts two to three hours) and requires time in the hospital, and, as doctors are prone to understate, "recovery time at home." In truth, recovery from this painful surgery can take 5 to 7 days in the hospital (depending on your doctor and hospital plan) and 8 to 10 weeks of recovery at home.[83] For some, recovery can take as long as 6 months.

All patients go home with a catheter in place to continually drain urine into a special bag. Even when the catheter is removed, most men continue to have poor urinary control in the beginning and require some form of protection, such as diapers or pads. Permanent urinary control problems will plague about 10 percent of men having a radical prostatectomy.

In his forthright book *Man to Man: Surviving Prostate Cancer*, Michael Korda, then editor-in-chief of Simon & Schuster, describes in vivid detail the personal indignities of prostate cancer; his battle with incontinence following a radical prostatectomy; and the surgical and postsurgical decisions and "goof-ups" by various members of his medical team that cause, among other complications, unremitting, excruciating pain for 24 hours, and possibly long-term, if not lasting, potency problems.[84]

All this after Korda, who had choices many of us don't have, had opted for the best of everything: a top hospital and the superstar surgeon who had developed a highly touted nerve-sparing, potency-saving surgery. However, this "superstar surgeon" mistakenly cut the nerves on one side of Korda's prostate without even informing him (he learned about it from another doctor weeks later). Any man who has prostate cancer, and especially those who have difficulty discussing the situation with others, should read Korda's informative book.

In addition to incontinence and impotence, other major disadvantages of a radical prostatectomy include blood loss and surgical complications. The surgery carries with it an average blood loss of greater than one unit of blood, extending up to as much as three or four units, so doctors usually must postpone surgery until the patient has been able to give the required number of pints of his own blood. Factors influencing blood loss include the size of the prostate and the anesthetic used. Patients under general anesthesia usually lose more blood than those who undergo epidural anesthesia.[85] In one study, low blood loss was significantly related to fewer complications after surgery.[86]

As with all surgeries, complications such as pain, infection, anesthetic problems, blood clots, heart problems, and even death can occur. No one ever expects that this simple listing, told almost casually to them by their surgeon, will happen to them—but it can. Unique to prostatectomy are injury to the rectum and scarring of the tissue used to make the new connection between the bladder and the urethra once the prostate has been removed.

ADVANCED THERAPIES

Where the cancer has spread (metastasized), the treatment choice will have to be one that affects the entire body, not just the prostate, because removing the prostate will not eliminate the cancer. Standard chemotherapy is unsuccessful in fighting prostate cancer—it wastes time and money, doesn't improve survival rates, and has debilitating side effects. That leaves radiation and hormonal therapies.

RADIATION THERAPY

External beam radiation therapy—a series of exposures over several weeks to a finely focused X-ray beam—can potentially cure prostate cancer in the early stages, although a research study conducted at

> *The appropriate candidate for radiation is a man*
> *who has a life expectancy of 10 years or more, and*
> *although he has a high-grade cancer, wants to avoid*
> *surgery yet wants to receive some kind of treatment.*
> *He must also be prepared to accept the uncertainty*
> *about the possible persistence of cancer.*[87]

Stanford University indicated that it was effective in only 20 percent of those receiving radiation. The remaining 75 to 80 percent of patients had an average doubling time of 15 months for Stage B cancer and 7 months for Stage C cancer, indicating the possibility that irradiation converted the cancer into a faster-growing one.[88] Radiation therapy is used also to palliate metastases to the bone; that is, to diminish pain and to lessen the likelihood of bone fractures.

External beam therapy is by far the simplest of prostate cancer therapies to administer (it involves no surgery, no anesthesia, and no blood loss) and consists of radiation aimed at the prostate from many different angles over a six- to seven-week period. Treatments usually last about 15 minutes and are administered five days a week.

The major disadvantage of this treatment is that the cancer is left in place, and doctors can never be quite sure that the amount of radiation delivered is enough to cure the cancer. Recent studies using transrectal ultrasound-guided biopsies showed residual tumor in 80 to 93 percent of patients two years after radiation treatment.[89] Another disadvantage is that tumors with ill-defined margins may not be adequately irradiated.

It is typical that at some time during the radiation treatment, a man will develop inflammation of the bladder or rectum, with diarrhea and urinary urgency, which may be serious enough to cause

treatment to be temporarily interrupted. Periodic flare-ups of diarrhea may occur for years after the radiation.

Another common side effect of radiation is fatigue. Permanent
radiation injury to the bladder or rectum are also distinct possibilities, resulting in chronic pain or bleeding. Other side effects may be
loss of appetite, nausea, vomiting, or symptoms of cystitis (frequency, urgency, and painful urination).

Most doctors will say politely that difficulty with erections can
occur in "a number of patients" who were having no problems
before radiation. At least one doctor is brave enough to state that
long-term effects include sexual impotence in 40 to 75 percent of
the men having external-beam radiation,[90] while Dr. Stephen Rous
estimates the figure to be 50 percent.[91] The impotence can take as
long as two years after treatment to show up. Dr. Rous suspects it is
related to the effects of the radiation on the blood vessels supplying
the spongy parts within the penis.[92] One European study documented the fact that radiotherapy of the prostate leads to more significant morbidity in patients than was generally anticipated by
doctors.[93]

At present, implantation of dozens of radioactive seeds into the
prostate (called interstitial brachytherapy) and cryotherapy, or freezing of the prostate, are being investigated as potential treatments.[94]
Both techniques have been around for 30 or 40 years although, as
you might suspect, they were originally more crude. In the 1970s,
implantation was done "freehand," and the results were not particularly encouraging.

Cryotherapy first involved open surgery so that liquid nitrogen
could be placed directly into the prostate cancer. Today both brachytherapy and cryotherapy involve using ultrasound as a guide to placing the implants or the cryotherapy needles. While both techniques
are now less invasive than surgery, thanks to technical advances,

they are not without their risks also, and no long-range studies yet exist to show that the treatments can, in fact, cure cancer.

Preliminary results of 55 men with localized prostate cancer proven by biopsy who underwent two different techniques of cryosurgery at Allegheny General Hospital in Pittsburgh, Pennsylvania, between June 1, 1990, and May 1, 1992, did show that for the 23 patients who had an associated biopsy at three-months follow-up, 19 of the men (82.6 percent) had no residual disease. Four (17.4 percent), did show positive results of prostate cancer. Although there were no deaths associated with the procedure, complications included freezing of the rectum in four patients, which resulted in urethrorectal fistula (the development of an abnormal passage) in two patients and the sloughing of prostatic urethral tissue in three patients. Of the 20 patients on which there was prepotency and postpotency data, 14 were potent before cryosurgery and six were not. Following the procedure, five of the 14 patients retained their potency; nine did not.[95]

HORMONAL THERAPY

Because the growth of prostate cancer cells is stimulated by the male hormone testosterone, hormone treatments to lower or shut down the production of testosterone may sometimes be another treatment option. First begun in the 1940s, hormonal treatments are usually used to slow the progression once the cancer has spread, or if it cannot be completely eradicated by surgery or radiation therapy.

Hormonal therapy is also sometimes used to shrink tumors prior to surgery, but it is never a curative option because prostate cancers contain androgen-independent (androgens are male sex hormones) or "insensitive" cells that are able to continue growing without testosterone. After an initial reduction in the tumor, the therapy may become ineffective within two or three years, and the cancer may again begin to grow (doctors call this the "hormonally refractory state"). For this reason, hormone therapy is not considered a viable alternative to surgery for men with reasonable life expectancies.

Hormone therapy should not be ignored, however, as a possibility for a spreading cancer, since it sometimes achieves a spectacular and long-lasting remission.[96] If hormonal therapy is started at the time of metastases to the bones, about 10 percent of patients will live at least 10 more years, 31 percent will live 5 more years, but 50 percent will live only 3 more years.[97]

Hormonal therapy is typically administered either by a monthly shot of medications (Lupron and Zoladex) that interfere with the production of androgens, or by surgical removal of the testicles, called an orchiectomy. Hormonal therapy is frequently the therapy of choice after other types of treatment have failed, although on occasion it may be a first choice.

Because the adrenal glands produce the hormone DHEA, which can be converted to testosterone, some testosterone usually remains in the body despite the administration of Lupron, so a second drug (a flutamide called Eulexin) is frequently given. The typical dose is two capsules taken orally every eight hours. This combined treatment—called a complete or combined hormonal blockade (CHB)— began to be available in the early 1980s in Canada but was not approved by the FDA for use in the United States until 1989. CHB has a number of side effects, including hot flashes, nausea, anemia, and complete sexual impotency.[98]

In the past, androgen deprivation therapy was used only as a palliative measure. A more recent approach combines radiation with hormonal therapy. An eight-year study reported in a 1997 issue of the *New England Journal of Medicine* followed 401 men in the age range of 51 to 80 years (median age, 71 years) who had "locally advanced prostate cancer"; that is, the cancer had spread outside the prostate but not to distant parts of the body. The study compared the effects of radiation therapy alone with the effects of radiation therapy combined with the simultaneous administration of goserelin (Zoladex) every four weeks. The statistically significant results showed that 62 percent of the men given radiation therapy alone survived for at least five years. The five-year survival rate climbed to 70 percent for the combined radiation-Zoladex group. Also significant was the proportion of surviving patients who were free of disease at five years: 85 percent in the combined treatment group compared to 48 percent in the radiotherapy-alone group.[99]

A new and promising technique of medical hormone therapy (LHRH therapy) stops the body's production of testosterone via monthly injections to control the production of the luteinizing hormone-releasing hormone. Frequently it is combined with oral antiandrogen medication to block the testosterone from the adrenal gland.[100]

According to the Pharmaceutical Research and Manufacturer's of America, about 25 pharmaceuticals currently in various stages of development or clinical trial may have value in the treatment of prostate cancer. Suramin, presently in clinical trials, is being considered for the management of patients with advanced prostate cancer for whom standard hormonal therapies have failed. Bicalutamide (brand name Casodex), and nilutamide (Anandron) are new antiandrogen drugs, believed to have similar clinical effects to flutamide. They already are available in other countries.[102]

The United States National Cancer Institute Intergroup Study #0036 demonstrated that the overall survival for patients with combined treatment, compared to those receiving single LHRH-agonist therapy, was an increase of about seven months. A subgroup of patients with minimal disease and good performance status achieved a 61-month median survival time, compared to 41 months in similar patients receiving only one medication.[101]

Whether or not you must undertake hormonal therapy, be prepared for the fact that you may not receive adequate or correct information about its effects. There is growing awareness that health care professionals often do not correctly recognize a patient's subjective morbidity (feelings about a disease). When 86 European urologists who were attending two scientific meetings were asked to complete questionnaires about their quality of life—imagining that they had stable prostate cancer and had been undergoing androgen deprivation (hormonal therapy) for at least one year—the doctors *underestimated* the disturbance of sexual life and the effects of fatigue and hot flashes, compared with questionnaires completed by 112 men who had actually undergone androgen deprivation. On the other hand, the doctors *overestimated* the impairment of quality of life and psychological distress experienced by these patients.[103]

ACTIONS TO TAKE AFTER A DIAGNOSIS

If you are diagnosed with prostate cancer, to paraphrase the poet Dylan Thomas, "do not go gently" into the first treatment or surgery your doctor recommends. Seek out at least one, and possibly two, other opinions from doctors not affiliated with your own.

Inform yourself, inform yourself, inform yourself. You are the one who—ultimately—will make the choice about your care. Find out all you can about your disorder, what stage it is in, and what the probabilities are for it to spread outside the prostate (unless it has already). Read the books referred to in this chapter.

Contact the American Cancer Society and/or the hospital in which your doctor practices to learn whether they have a prostate cancer group. Find one, go to the meetings, and talk to men who have had prostate cancer and prostatectomies. Trust us: they will know more about the actual long-term consequences of suggested surgery than your doctor will tell you. By that, we mean, that your doctor certainly will tell you some of the probabilities of his proposed treatment—he would be medically remiss if he did not—but he will present them fairly straightforwardly, objectively, and reassuringly (". . . and if this does occur, there are things we can do about it"); whereas, the men in the groups live with the results day-to-day. They also are likely to have strong opinions about the surgeon and the hospital you are considering, and their subjectivity will have to be balanced with the other information you are acquiring.

If you are on the Internet, there are a number of health sites that have up-to-date information on prostate cancer (such as The Prostate Cancer InfoLink at http://www.comed.com/Prostate), plus "chat groups" of men who have been diagnosed in various stages of prostate cancer, or who have had a prostatectomy. Learn about their concerns; ask questions of your own.

If you have decided on surgery, study the credentials of your surgeon; that is, how many times and with what success has he done the surgery you are contemplating. Tell him your fears; ask him your questions. If you don't like his answers, or he won't discuss his numbers regarding surgery, find someone you can trust and that you will have confidence in. As Michael Korda cautions, remember that "surgery is a job like any other, and it's up to him to convince you he's the right man for you."[104]

8

Conclusion

A
lthough the symptoms of benign prostatic hyperplasia often begin to occur when a man reaches his 40s or 50s, BPH is a disease definitely associated with aging, and in the United States, the elderly are the fastest-growing segment of the population. In 1990 there were 33 million Americans over the age of 65 years. By the year 2000 that number is expected to swell to 37 million.[1] As a result, more and more men will experience BPH and seek treatment for it.

While in years past the diagnosis of BPH had been assigned to nearly all men who presented a rather loosely defined set of symptoms known generally as "prostatism," medical researchers and urologists are making considerable efforts to sharpen their diagnostic focus and improve the precision of their terminology. They are attempting to distinguish between the lower urinary tract symptoms that are so common in aging men—and women, for that matter—and those that are a specific result of an enlarged prostate.

With those ends in mind, many in the medical field have also turned their attention toward technological and pharmaceutical advances that will assist in alleviating the symptoms of BPH. Fortunately, new methods for decreasing the distress of BPH continue to be steadily developed or improved.

Only two classes of drugs, alpha-adrenergic blockers and 5-alpha-reductase inhibitors, are currently used in the United States to treat mild to moderate symptoms. Both have serious side effects that often cause men to stop taking them. Patient compliance is considered a major problem in the pharmaceutical treatment of BPH. While treatments with an alpha-blocker can produce rapid relief, the results are not as good with surgery, and adverse effects—such as dizziness upon rising—may be problematic for many men. The slow onset of finasteride means that its effects may not become apparent until after at least six months—or possibly a year—of therapy.

In the near future, physicians will almost certainly be exposed to new drug developments for the treatment of BPH (different 5-alpha-reductase enzyme inhibitors and better alpha adrenoceptor blockers)—all of which will have to prove their value in the kinds of long-term, placebo-controlled, double-blind clinical trials described in Chapter 1 as constituting good research. Long-term studies are currently underway to determine whether combining the two types of drugs will prove more effective than using either alone.[2]

At least one clinical trial conducted by the Department of Veterans Affairs suggested that more men in a terazosin/finasteride combination therapy withdrew from the study because of adverse events than those in one or more of the monotherapy groups.[3] In addition, no research has been completed to indicate how frequently patients require surgery after several years of drug therapy.

Urologic procedures continue to be the money-slashing targets of governmental agencies and third-party payors, in order to reduce overall health care expenditure. Doctors are currently reviewing the safety and cost savings of performing transurethral resection of the prostate (TURP), the most commonly performed BPH surgery, as an outpatient procedure, allowing the patient to recover at home.[4]

While it is estimated that the annual savings to the health care system would be more than $3 billion per year, it must be carefully determined who the most appropriate patients are for TURP on an outpatient basis, and how this will psychologically and medically affect the patient.

Fortunately, one no longer has to wait for the completion of new technological developments or ongoing studies to resolve a BPH problem. We believe we have shown conclusively in this book that something *can* be done to relieve the uncomfortable and embarrassing symptoms of BPH, beyond waiting for new developments, undergoing surgery with its painful recovery time, or taking medications, all of which have discouraging side effects. The Prostate Cure, Cernitin, *already* holds the promise of symptom resolution. Cernitin works without either pain or side effects. It is safe and effective—a simple, desirable alternative to a painful or bleak future.

No longer will the afflicted have to get up several times during the night, or worry where bathrooms are along the route to work or in the places where they shop. Now it is possible to relieve not only BPH symptoms, but worries about them as well. By using Cernitin and incorporating the diet and exercise program and stress management techniques outlined in Chapters 5 and 6 of this book, the patient is well on his way to relief from the annoying symptoms of BPH.

In Chapter 2 we discussed the need to consult a doctor to determine that symptoms are, indeed, the result of benign prostatic hyperplasia and not some other disorder that can quickly be relieved or that requires a different kind of treatment.

Once the diagnosis of BPH has been established, you can embark on The Prostate Cure. By taking Cernitin and following our simple seven-point plan (outlined in Chapter 5), you join men all over the world who have experienced success using Cernitin to combat their prostatitis and BPH, and to reduce the possibility of a further increase in symptoms. Suddenly, you—not your enlarged prostate— are in charge of your health, happiness, and quality of life. And what could be better than that?

N O T E S

AUTHORS' NOTE

1. Boyarsky, S., G. Jones, D. F. Paulson, and G. R. Prout. A New Look at Bladder Neck Obstruction by the Food and Drug Administration Regulators: Guidelines for the Investigation of Benign Prostatic Hypertrophy. *Transactions of the American Association of Genito-urinary Surgeons*, 1977, 68, 29–32.

2. Barry, M. J., F. J. Fowler, Jr., M. P. O'Leary, R. C. Bruskewitz, H. L. Holtgrewe, W. K. Mebust, and A. T. Cockett. The American Urological Association Symptom Index for Benign Prostatic Hyperplasia. The Measurement Committee of the American Urological Association. *Journal of Urology*, 1992, 148, 1549–1557.

3. Roberts, R. G. BPH: New Guidelines Based on Symptoms and Patient Preference. The Agency for Health Care Policy and Research. *Geriatrics*, 1994, 49, 24–31.

4. Boyle, P. Cultural and Linguistic Validation of Questionnaires for Use in International Studies: The Nine-item BPH-specific Quality-of-Life Scale. *European Urology*, 1997, 32 (suppl. 2), 50–52.

5. Ibid.

CHAPTER 1: BENIGN PROSTATIC HYPERPLASIA (BPH): MEN'S SECRET DISEASE

1. Salcedo, H. *The Prostate. Facts and Misconceptions.* NY: A Birch Lane Press Book, 1993.

2. Kortt, M. A., and J. L. Bootman. The Economics of Benign Prostatic Hyperplasia Treatment: A Literature Review. *Clinical Therapeutics*, 1996, 18(6), 1227–1241.

3. Jacobsen, S. J., C. J. Girman, H. A. Guess, J. E. Oesterling, and M. M. Lieber. New Diagnostic and Treatment Guidelines for Benign Prostatic Hyperplasia.

Potential Impact in the United States. *Archives of Internal Medicine,* 13 March 1995, 155(5), 477–481.4. Oesterling, op. cit., p. 69.

4. Oesterling, op. cit., p. 69.

5. Oesterling, op. cit., p. 69.

6. Mindell, E. *Food as Medicine.* NY: A Fireside Book, 1994, p. 265.

7. Rous, S. N. *The Prostate Book.* Rev. ed. NY: W. W. Norton & Co., 1994, p. 87.

8. Rous, op. cit., p. 11.

9. Ibid.

10. Cited in Brown, D. J. *Herbal Prescriptions for Better Health: Your Everyday Guide to Prevention, Treatment, and Care.* Rocklan, CA: Prima Publishing Co., 1996.

11. Rous, op. cit., p. 19.

12. Buttyan, R., M.-W. Chen, and R. M. Levin. Animal Models of Bladder Outlet Obstruction and Molecular Insights into the Basis for the Development of Bladder Dysfunction. *European Urology,* 1997, 32 (suppl. 1), 32–39.

13. Salcedo, op. cit., p. 10.

14. Walsh, P. C., and J. F. Worthington. *The Prostate. A Guide for Men and the Women Who Love Them.* Baltimore and London: The Johns Hopkins University Press, 1995, p. 15.

15. Oesterling, J. E. Benign Prostatic Hyperplasia: A Review of Its Histogenesis and Natural History. *The Prostate Supplement,* 1996, 6, 67–73.

16. Rous, op. cit., p. 89.

17. Lawson, R. K. Role of Growth Factors in Benign Prostatic Hyperplasia. *European Urology,* 1997, 32 (suppl. 1), 22–27.

18. Salcedo, op. cit., p. 15.

19. Korda, M. *Man to Man: Surviving Prostate Cancer.* NY: Random House, 1996, p. 17.

20. Salcedo, op. cit., p. 15.

21. Rous, op. cit., p. 99.

22. Lawson, op. cit.

23. Korda, op. cit., p. 18

24. Salmans, S. *Prostate. Questions You Have . . . Answers You Need.* Allentown, PA: People's Medical Society, 1993, p. 20.

25. Rous, op. cit., p. 99.

26. Stewart, C. Prostatitis. *Emergency Medicine Clinics of North America,* Aug. 1988, 6(3), 391–402.

27. Ebeling, L. "Therapeutic Results of Defined Pollen-Extract in Patients with Chronic Prostatitis or BPH Accompanied by Chronic Prostatitis." In *Therapy of Prostatitis,* E. Schmiedt, J. E. Alken, and H. W. Bauer, eds. Munich: Zuckschwerdt Verlag, 1986, pp. 154–160.

28. Criste, G., D. Gray, and B. Gallo. Prostatitis: A Review of Diagnosis and Management. *Nurse Practitioner,* July 1994, 19(7), 32–33.

29. Ebeling, op. cit., p. 154.

30. Shortliffe, L. M. D. Prostatitis. *Primary Care,* 1985, 12(4), 787–794.

31. Moul, J. W. Prostatitis: Sorting Out the Different Causes. *Postgraduate Medicine,* Oct. 1993, 94(5), 191–194.

32. Walsh and Worthington, op. cit., p. 294.

33. Moul, op. cit.

34. Salmans, op. cit., p. 28.

35. Moul, op. cit.

36. Shortliffe, op. cit.

37. Stewart, op. cit.

38. Miller, H. C. Stress Prostatitis. *Urology,* Dec. 1988, 32(6), 507–510.

39. Salcedo, op. cit., p. 106.

40. Ibid.

41. Mene, M. P., P. C. Ginsberg, L. H. Finkelstein, S. J. Manfrey, L. Belkoff, F. Ogbolu, and D. Osborne. Transurethral Microwave Hyperthermia in the Treatment of Chronic Nonbacterial Prostatitis. *Journal of the American Osteopathic Association,* Jan. 1997, 97(1), 25–30.

42. Walsh and Worthington, op. cit., p. 280.

43. Rous, op. cit., pp. 73–74.

44. Moul, op. cit.

45. Salcedo, op. cit., pp. 106–107.

46. Shortliffe, op. cit.

47. Salcedo, op. cit., p. 107.

48. Servadio, C., and Z. Leib. Chronic Abacterial Prostatitis and Hyperthermia. A Possible New Treatment. *British Journal of Urology,* March 1991, 67(3), 308–311.

49. Kumon, H., N. Ono, S. Uno, T. Hayashi, K. Hata, T. Takenaka, T. Watanabe, and H. Ohmori. Transrectal Hyperthermia for the Treatment of Chronic Prostatitis. *Nippon Hinyokika Gakkai Zasshi,* Feb. 1993, 84(2), 265–271.

50. Nickel, J. C., and R. Sorensen. Transurethral Microwave Thermotherapy for

Nonbacterial Prostatitis: A Randomized Double-blind Sham Controlled Study Using New Prostatitis Specific Assessment Questionnaires. *Journal of Urology,* June 1996, 155(6), 1950–1954.

51. Ikeuchi, T., and H. Iguchi. Clinical Studies on Chronic Prostatitis and Prostatitis-like Syndrome (7). Electric Acupuncture Therapy for Intractable Cases of Chronic Prostatitis-like Syndrome. *Acta Urologica Japan,* July 1994, 40(7), 587–591.

52. Egan, K. J., and J. N. Krieger. *Clinical Journal of Pain,* Sept. 1994, 10(3), 218–226.

53. Berghuis, J. P., J. R. Heiman, I. Rothman, and R. E. Berger. Psychological and Physical Factors Involved in Chronic Idiopathic Prostatitis. *Journal of Psychosomatic Research,* Oct. 1996, 41(4), 313–325.

54. de la Rosette, J. J., M. C. Ruijgrok, J. M. Jeuken, H. F. Karthaus, and F. M. Debruyne. Personality Variables Involved in Chronic Prostatitis. *Urology,* Dec. 1993, 42(6), 654–662.

55. Wenninger, K., J. R. Heiman, I. Rothman, J. P. Berghuis, and R. E. Berger. Sickness Impact of Chronic Nonbacterial Prostatitis and Its Correlates. *Journal of Urology,* March 1996, 155(3), 965–968.

56. Egan, K. J., and J. N. Krieger. Chronic Abacterial Prostatitis—A Urological Chronic Pain Syndrome? *Pain,* Feb. 1997, 69(3), 213–218.

57. Ibid.

58. Krieger, J. N., K. J. Egan, S. O. Ross, R. Jacobs, R. E. Berger. Chronic Pelvic Pains Represent the Most Prominent Urogenital Symptoms of "Chronic Prostatitis." *Urology,* Nov. 1996, 48(5), 715–721.

59. Salmans, op. cit., p. 54.

60. Rous, op. cit., p. 12.

61. Salcedo, op. cit., p. 65.

62. Walsh and Worthington, op. cit., p. 14.

63. Salmans, op. cit., p. 43.

64. Ibid.

65. Weisser, H., and M. Krieg. Benign Prostatic Hyperplasia—The Outcome of Age-Induced Alteration of Androgen-Estrogen Balance? *Urologe A,* Jan. 1997, 36(1), 3–9.

66. The home page may be accessed on the Internet at http://www.niddk.gov/ niddk_homepage.html [no period].

67. Schachter, M. "The Male Andropause." Found on Health World Online at http://www.healthy.net/library/articles/schacter/andropas.d.htm.

68. Imperato-McGinley, J., L. Guerrero, T. Gautier, and R. E. Peterson. Steroid 5α-reductase Deficiency in Man: An Inherited Form of Male Pseudohermaphroditism. *Science,* 1974, 186, 1213–1215. For the report of the second group, see Walsh, P. C., J. D. Madden, M. J. Harrod, J. L. Goldstein, P. C. Macdonald, and J. D. Wilson. Familial Incomplete Male Pseudohermaphroditism Type 2. Decreased Dihydrotestosterone Formation in Pseudovaginal Perineoscrotal Hypospadias. *New England Journal of Medicine,* 1974, 291, 944–949.

69. Monda, and Oesterling, op. cit.

70. Thigpen, A. E., D. L. Davis, A. Milatovich, B. B. Mendonca, J. Imperato-McGinley, J. E. Griffin, U. Francke, J. D. Wilson, and D. W. Russell. Molecular Genetics of Steroid 5α-reductase 2 Deficiency. *Journal of Clinical Investigation,* 1992, 90, 799–809.

71. Imperato-McGinley, J., T. Gautier, K. Zirinsky, T. Hom, O. Palomo, E. Stein, E. D. Vaughan, J. A. Markisz, E. Ramirez de Arellano, and E. Kazam. Prostate Visualization Studies in Males Homozygous and Heterozygous for 5 Alpha-reductase Deficiency. *Journal of Clinical Endocrinology and Metabolism,* 1992, 75, 1022–1026.

72. Stoner, E. 5α-reductase Inhibitors/Finasteride. *The Prostate Supplement,* 1996, 6, 82–87.

73. Ibid.

CHAPTER 2: STANDARD NON-ORAL APPROACHES TO TREATING BPH

1. Collins, M. M., M. J. Barry, L. Bin, R. G. Roberts, J. E. Oesterling, and F. J. Fowler. Diagnosis and Treatment of Benign Prostatic Hyperplasia. Practice Patterns of Primary Care Physicians. *Journal of General Internal Medicine,* April 1997, 12(4), 224–229.

2. Rous, op. cit., p. 190.

3. Nensink, H. Evaluation of Benign Prostatic Hyperplasia Treatments: How Can We Improve the Outcome Measures and Success Criteria? *European Urology,* 1997, 32 (suppl. 2), 38–41.

4. Blute, M. L. Transurethral Microwave Thermotherapy: Minimally Invasive Therapy for Benign Prostatic Hyperplasia. *Urology,* 1997, 50(2), 163–166.

5. Oesterling, op. cit., p. 70.

6. Barry, M. J. Epidemiology and Natural History of Benign Prostatic Hyperplasia. *Urology Clinics of North America,* Aug. 1990, 17(3), 495–507.

7. Kawachi, I., M. J. Barry, E. Giovannucci, E. B. Rimm, G. A. Colditz, M. J. Stampfer, and W. C. Willett. The Impact of Different Therapies on Symptoms of Benign Prostatic Hyperplasia: A Prospective Study. *Clinical Therapeutics,* November 1996, 18(6), 1118–1127.

8. Flood, A. B., N. A. Black, K. McPherson, J. Smith, and G. Williams. *Archives of Internal Medicine,* July 1992, 152(7), 1507–1512.

9. Eri, L. M., and K. J. Tveter. Treatment of Benign Prostatic Hyperplasia. A Pharmacoeconomic Perspective. *Drugs and Aging,* Feb. 1997, 10(2), 107–118.

10. Holtgrewe, H. L. "Report on the Economics of BPH." In *Proceedings of the 3rd International Conference on BPH.* A. T. K. Crockett, S. Khoury, Y. Aso, C. Chatelain, L. Denis, K. Griffiths, and G. Murphy, eds. Monaco, 1995, 226–228.

11. Tammela, T. Benign Prostatic Hyperplasia. Practical Treatment Guidelines. *Drugs & Aging,* May 1997, 10(5), 349–366.

12. Ball, A. J., R. C. Feneley, and P. H. Abrams. The Natural History of Untreated "Prostatism." *British Journal of Urology,* 1981, 53, 613–616.

13. Tan, H. Y., W. C. Choo, C. Archibald, and K. Esuvaranathan. A Community Based Study of Prostatic Symptoms in Singapore. *Journal of Urology,* March 1997, 157(3), 890–893.

14. Peters, T. J., J. L. Donovan, H. E. Kay, P. Abrams, J. J. de la Rosette, D. Porru, and J. W. Thuroff. The International Continence Society "Benign Prostatic Hyperplasia" Study: The Bothersomeness of Urinary Symptoms. *Journal of Urology,* March 1997, 157(3), 885–889.

15. Mensink, H. Evaluation of Benign Prostatic Hyperplasia Treatments: How Can We Improve the Outcome Measures and Success Criteria? *European Urology,* 1997, 32 (suppl. 2), 38–41.

16. Tammela, op. cit., May 1997, 10(5), 349–366.

17. Rous, op. cit., pp. 89, 155.

18. Wein, A. J. Assessing Treatment Results in Benign Prostatic Hyperplasia *Urological Clinics of North America,* 1995, 22, 345–355.

19. Lawson, R. K. Role of Growth Factors in Benign Prostatic Hyperplasia. *European Urology,* 1997, 32 (suppl. 1), 22–27.

20. Carter, H. B., and D. S. Coffey. The Prostate: An Increasing Medical Problem. *The Prostate,* 1990, 16, 39–49.

21. Margolis, S., and H. B. Carter. *Prostate Disorders.* The 1997 Johns Hopkins white paper. Baltimore, Maryland: The Johns Hopkins Medical Institutions, 1997, p. 15.

22. Ibid.

23. Tammela, op. cit.

24. Lowe, F. C., R. L. McDaniel, J. J. Chmiel, and A. L. Hillman. Economic Modeling to Assess the Costs of Treatment with Finasteride, Terazosin, and Transurethral Resection of the Prostate for Men with Moderate to Severe Symptoms of Benign Prostatic Hyperplasia. *Urology,* 1995, 46, 477–483.

25. D'Ancona, F. C. H., E. A. E. Francisca, F. M. J. Debruyne, and J. J. M. C. H. de la Rosette. High-energy Transurethral Microwave Thermotherapy in Men with Lower Urinary Tract Symptoms. *Journal of Endourology,* Aug. 1997, 11(4), 285–289.

26. Desgrandchamps, F. Clinical Relevance of Growth Factor Antagonists in the Treatment of Benign Prostatic Hyperplasia. *European Urology,* 1997, 32 (suppl. 1), 28–31.

27. Rous, op. cit., p. 158.

28. Tammela, op. cit., 1977.

29. Margolis and Carter, op. cit., p. 17.

30. Hartung, R. Updated Patient Information for Treatment of Benign Prostatic Hyperplasia: A Permanent Challenge. *European Urology,* 1997, 32 (suppl. 2), 42–44. See also Tammela, T., op. cit.

31. Horninger, W., H. Unterlechner, H. Strasser, and G. Bartsch. Transurethral Prostatectomy: Mortality and Morbidity. *The Prostate,* 1996, 28, 195–200.

32. Wasson, J. H., D. J. Reda, R. C. Bruskewitz, et al. A Comparison of Transurethral Surgery with Watchful Waiting for Moderate Symptoms of Benign Prostatic Hyperplasia. *New England Journal of Medicine,* 1995, 332, 75–79. Cited in Tammela, T., op. cit.

33. Cattolica, E. V., S. Sidney, and M. C. Sadler. The Safety of Transurethral Prostatectomy: A Cohort Study of Mortality in 9,416 Men. *Journal of Urology,* July 1997, 158(1), 102–104.

34. Walsh and Worthington, op. cit., p. 239.

35. Blute, op. cit., p. 165.

36. Ibid., p. 164.

37. Hallin, Anders, R. Stege, Tomas Berlin, and K. Carlström. Transurethral Microwave Thermotherapy in Symptomatic Benign Prostatic Hyperplasia: A Possible Association Between Androgen Status and Treatment Result? *The Prostate,* 1997, 33, 13–17.

38. de la Rosette, J. J., F. C. D'Ancona, and F. M. Debruyne. Current Status of Thermotherapy of the Prostate. *Journal of Urology,* Feb. 1997, 157(2), 430–438.

39. Blute, op. cit., p. 164.

40. Cher, D. J., and L. A. Lenert. "New Treatments for Benign Prostatic Hypertrophy—A Decision Model." Paper presented at the Society for Medical Decision Making, 13–16, Oct. 1996, Toronto, Canada.

41. Ahmed, M., T. Bell, W. T. Lawrence, J. P. Ward, and G. M. Watson. Transurethral Microwave Thermotherapy (Prostatron Version 2.5) Compared with Transurethral Resection of the Prostate for the Treatment of Benign Prostatic Hyperplasia: A Randomized, Controlled, Parallel Study. *British Journal of Urology,* Feb. 1997, 79(2), 181–185.

42. Note that Hernando Salcedo in his book on the prostate (*The Prostate. Facts and Misconceptions.* NY: Carol Publishing Group, 1993, p. 50) remarks that BPH is a disease characterized by spontaneous improvement, so that it is not surprising that in many studies improvement is noticed in both treated and placebo controls after a short period of time. "This makes evaluation of the effect of the treatment very difficult," he concludes.

43. Nawrocki, J. D., T. J. Bell, W. T. Lawrence, and J. P. Ward. A Randomized Controlled Trial of Transurethral Microwave Thermotherapy. *British Journal of Urology,* March 1997, 79(3), 389–393.

44. Ahmed, Bell, Lawrence, et al., op. cit.

45. D'Ancona, Francisca, Debruyne, et al., op. cit.

46. D'Ancona, F. C., E. A. Francisca, W. P. Witjes, L. Welling, F. M. Debruyne, and J. J. de la Rosette. High Energy Thermotherapy Versus Transurethral Resection in the Treatment of Benign Prostatic Hyperplasia: Results of a Prospective Randomized Study with One Year Followup. *Journal of Urology,* July 1997, 158(1), 120–125.

47. Blute, op. cit., p. 166.

48. Naslund, M. J. Transurethral Needle Ablation of the Prostate. *Urology,* 1997, 50(2), 167–172.

49. Naslund, op. cit., p. 171.

50. Hartung, op. cit., p. 44.

51. Naslund, op. cit., p. 170.

52. Ramon, J., T. H. Lynch, I. Eardley, P. Ekman, J. Frick, A. Jungwirth, M. Pillai, P. Wiklund, B. Goldwasser, and J. M. Fitzpatrick. Transurethral Needle Ablation of the Prostate for the Treatment of Benign Prostatic Hyperplasia: A Collaborative Multicentre Study. *British Journal of Urology,* July 1997, 80(1), 128–134.

53. Campo, B., F. Berhamaschi, P. Corrada, and G. Ordesi. Transurethral Needle Ablation (TUNA) of the Prostate: A Clinical and Urodynamic Evaluation. *Urology,* June 1997, 49(6), 847–850.

54. Margolis and Carter, op. cit., p. 17.

55. Walsh and Worthington, op. cit., pp. 252–253.

56. Mulligan, E. D., T. H. Lynch, D. Mulvin, D. Greene, J. M. Smith, and J. M. Fitzpatrick. High-intensity Focused Ultrasound in the Treatment of Benign Prostatic Hyperplasia. *British Journal of Urology,* Feb. 1997, 79(2), 177–180.

57. Sullivan, L. D., M. G. McLoughlin, L. G. Goldenberg, M. E. Gleave, and K. W. Marich. Early Experience with High-intensity Focused Ultrasound for the Treatment of Benign Prostatic Hypertrophy. *British Journal of Urology,* Feb. 1997, 79(2), 172–176.

58. Walsh and Worthington, op. cit., p. 248.

59. Salcedo, op. cit., p. 55.

60. Ibid., p. 54.

61. Dinsmoor, R. Benign Prostate Disease. Looking at Surgery in a New Light. *Harvard Health Letter,* Dec. 1993, 19(2), 6–8.

62. Chen, S. S., A. W. Chiu, A. T. Lin, K. K. Chen, and L. S. Chang. Clinical Outcome at 3 Months After Transurethral Vaporization of Prostate for Benign Prostatic Hyperplasia. *Urology,* Aug. 1997, 50(2), 235–238.

63. Tuttle, J. P. VLAP Is Quicker, Less Painful, and Cheaper than TURP. *Clinical Laser Monthly,* 1993, 11, 187–189.

64. Sanders, J. A., and J. H. Reese. The Use of Lasers as an Alternative Treatment for Patients with Benign Prostatic Hyperplasia. *Journal of Urological Nursing,* 1994, 13, 656–659.

65. Dinsmoor, op. cit.

66. Furuya, S., H. Ogura, Y. Tanaka, T. Tsukamoto, N. Daikuzono, and M. L. Liong. Transurethral Balloon Laser Thermotherapy for Urinary Retention in

Patients with Benign Prostatic Hyperplasia Who Are at High Surgical Risk. *International Journal of Urology,* May 1997, 4(3), 265–268.

67. Anonymous. Enlarged Prostate: Evaluating Your Options. "Health After 50" column. *Johns Hopkins Medical Letter,* April 1995, 7(2), 4–6.

68. Margolis and Carter, op. cit., p. 17.

69. Kortt and Bootman, op. cit., p. 1230.

70. Margolis and Carter, op. cit., p. 18.

71. Hollander, J. B., and A. C. Diokno. Prostatism: Benign Prostatic Hyperplasia. *Urological Clinics of North America,* Feb. 1996, 23(1), 75–86.

72. You can reach the Urology home page of Columbia-Presbyterian Prostate Center at http://cpmcnet.columbia.edu/dept/urology/bph.html.

73. Kaplan, S. A., and A. E. Te. Transurethral Electrovaporization of the Prostate (TVP): A Novel Method of Treating Men with Benign Prostatic Hyperplasia. *Urology,* 1995, 45, 566–573.

74. Thomas, K. J., A. J. Cornaby, M. Hammadeh, T. Philip, and P. N. Matthews. Transurethral Vaporization of the Prostate: A Promising New Technique. *British Journal of Urology,* Feb. 1997, 79(2), 186–189.

75. Tammela, op. cit.

76. Ito, T., K. Fujita, T. Hori, and H. Sakagami. Clinical Study of Intraurethral Stent for Patients with Benign Prostatic Hypertrophy with 1-Year Follow Up. *Acta Urologica Japan,* 1994, 40, 593–595.

CHAPTER 3: THE ALTERNATIVES TO SURGERY

1. Desgrandchamps, F. Clinical Relevance of Growth Factor Antagonists in the Treatment of Benign Prostatic Hyperplasia. *European Urology,* 1997, 32 (suppl. 1), 28–31.

2. Blomqvist, P., A. Ekbom, P. Carlsson, C. Ahlstrand, and J. E. Johansson. Benign Prostatic Hyperplasia in Sweden 1987 to 1994: Changing Patterns of Treatment, Changing Patterns of Costs. *Urology,* Aug. 1997, 50(2), 214–219.

3. Barry, M. J., F. J. Fowler, Jr., L. Bin, and J. E. Oesterling. A Nationwide Survey of Practicing Urologists: Current Management of Benign Prostatic Hyperplasia and Clinically Localized Prostate Cancer. *Journal of Urology,* Aug. 1997, 158(2), 488–491.

4. Roehrborn, C. G., J. E. Oesterling, S. Auerbach, S. A. Kaplan, L. K. Lloyd, D. E.

Milam, and R. J. Padley. The Hytrin Community Assessment Trial Study: A One-year Study of Terazosin versus Placebo in the Treatment of Men with Symptomatic Benign Prostatic Hyperplasia. HYCAT Investigator Group. *Urology,* Feb. 1996, 47(2), 159–168.

5. Bernier, P. A., and C. G. Roehrborn. Recent Trials for Medical Treatment of Benign Prostatic Hyperplasia. *Infections in Urology,* 1997, 19(4), 118–125.

6. Ibid.

7. Consumers Union. *Complete Drug Reference.* Yonkers, NY: Consumers Union, 1997, p. 1540.

8. Lepor, H., S. A. Kaplan, I. Klimberg, D. F. Mobley, A. Fawzy, M. Gaffney, K. Ice, N. Dias, and the Multicenter Study Group. Doxazosin for Benign Prostatic Hyperplasia: Long-Term Efficacy and Safety in Hypertensive and Normotensive Patients. *Journal of Urology,* Feb. 1997, 157(2), 525–530.

9. Ibid.

10. Tammela, op. cit.

11. Ibid., p. 361.

12. Ekman, P., J. T. Andersen, and H. Wolf. Finasteride in the Treatment of Benign Prostatic Hyperplasia. *Acta Urologica Belgica,* March 1996, 64(1), ix–xii.

13. Brawley, O. W., L. G. Ford, I. M. Thompson, J. A. Perlman, and B. S. Kramer. 5-alpha-reductase Inhibition and Prostate Cancer Prevention. *Cancer Epidemiology Biomarkers and Prevention,* 1994, 3, 177–182.

14. Stoner, E. 5 Alpha-reductase Inhibitors/Finasteride. *The Prostate Supplement,* 1996, 6, 82–87.

15. Is Proscar Right for You? Health After 50 column. Johns Hopkins Medical Letter, Sept. 1992, 4(7), 1–2.

16. Keetch, D. W. Medical Therapy for Benign Prostatic Hyperplasia. *Infections in Urology,* 1997, 19(2), 54–60.

17. Gormley, G. J., E. Stoner, R. C. Bruskewitz, J. Imperato-McGinley, P. C. Walsh, J. D. McConnell, G. L. Andriole, J. Geller, B. R. Bracken, and J. S. Tenover. The Effect of Finasteride in Men with Benign Prostatic Hyperplasia. *New England Journal of Medicine,* 1992, 327, 1185–1191.

18. Consumers Union, op. cit., p. 797. See also Gormley, G. J., E. Stoner, R. C. Bruskewitz, et al., op. cit.

19. Tenover, J. L., G. A. Pagano, A. S. Morton, C. L. Liss, and C. A. Byrnes. Efficacy and Tolerability of Finasteride in Symptomatic Benign Prostatic Hyperpla-

sia: A Primary Care Study. Primary Care Investigator Study Group. *Clinical Therapeutics*, March 1997, 19(2), 243–258.

20. Tammela, op. cit.

21. Keetch, op. cit.

22. Oesterling, J. E., J. Roy, A. Agha, T. Shown, T. Krarup, T. Johansen, M. Lagerkvist, G. Gormley, M. Bach, and J. Waldstreicher. Biologic Variability of Prostate-Specific Antigen and Its Usefulness as a Marker for Prostate Cancer: Effects of Finasteride. The Finasteride PSA Study Group. *Urology*, July 1997, 59(1), 13–18.

23. Keetch, op. cit.

24. Ibid.

25. Eri and Tveter, op. cit.

26. Andersen, J. T., J. C. Nickel, V. R. Marshall, C. C. Schulman, and P. Boyle. Finasteride Significantly Reduces Acute Urinary Retention and Need for Surgery in Patients with Symptomatic Benign Prostatic Hyperplasia. *Urology*, Jan. 1997, 49(6), 839–845.

27. Lee, M., and R. Sharifi. Benign Prostatic Hyperplasia: Diagnosis and Treatment Guideline. *Annals of Pharmacotherapy*, April 1997, 31(4), 481–486.

28. Consumers Union, op. cit., p. 796.

29. Cooner, W. H. Y., B. R. Mosley, C. L. Rutherford, Jr., J. H. Beard, H. S. Pond, R. B. Bass, Jr., and W. J. Terry. Clinical Application of TRUS and PSA in the Search for Prostate Cancer. *Journal of Urology*, 1988, 139, 758–761.

30. Thompson, I. M., C. A. Coltman, Jr., and J. Crowley. Chemoprevention of Prostate Cancer: The Prostate Cancer Prevention Trial. *The Prostate*, 1997, 33, 217–221.

31. Ibid.

32. Nakayama, O., J. Hirosumi, N. Chica, S. Takahashi, K. Sawada, H. Kojo, and Y. Notsu. FR146687, a Novel Steroid 5-Alpha-reductase Inhibitor: In Vitro and In Vivo Effects on Prostates. *The Prostate*, 1 June 1997, 31(4), 241–249.

33. Inami, M., I. Kawamura, Y. Nnaoe, S. Tsujimoto, T. Mizota, T. Manda, and K. Shimomura. Effects of a New Non-steroidal 5 Alpha-reductase Inhibitor, FK143, on the Prostate Gland in Beagle Dogs. *Japanese Journal of Pharmacology*, June 1997, 74(2), 187–194.

34. Bramson, H. N., D. Hermann, K. W. Batchelor, F. W. Lee, M. K. James, and S. V. Frye. Unique Preclinical Characteristics of GG745, a Potent Dual Inhibitor of

5 AR. *Journal of Pharmacology and Experimental Therapeutics,* Sept. 1997, 282(3), 1496–1502.

35. Minter, S. *The Healing Garden.* Boston: Charles E. Tuttle Co., Inc., 1993, p. 9.

36. Ibid., p. 12.

37. American Medical Association. *Reader's Guide to Alternative Health Methods.* Milwaukee, WI: American Medical Association, 1993, p. 74.

38. Lukacs, B. Using a Large Clinical Database to Assess the Effectiveness of Alfuzosin. *European Urology,* 1997, 32 (suppl. 2), 45–47.

39. Dreikorn, K., and P. S. Schonhofer. Status of Phytotherapeutic Drugs in Treatment of Benign Prostatic Hyperplasia. *Urologe Ausgabe A,* March 1995, 34(2), 119–129.

40. Bracher, F. Phytotherapy of Benign Prostatic Hyperplasia. *Urologe Ausgabe A,* Jan. 1997, 36(1), 10–17.

41. Weisser, H., S. Tunn, B. Behnke, and M. Krieg. Effects of the Sabal serrulata Extract IDS89 and Its Subfractions on 5α-Reductase Activity in Human Benign Prostatic Hyperplasia. *The Prostate,* 1996, 28, 300–306.

42. Breu, W., M. Hagenlocher, K. Redl, G. Tittel, F. Stadler, and H. Watner. Anti-inflammatory Activity of Sabal Fruit Extracts Prepared with Supercritical Carbon Dioxide. In Vitro Antagonists of Cyclooxygenase and 5-Lipoxygenase Metabolism. *Arzneimittelforschung,* April 1992, 42(4), 547–551.

43. Weiner, M. A., and J. Weiner. *Herbs That Heal.* Mill Valley, CA: Quantum Books, 1994, pp. 290–291.

44. Carraro, J.-C., J.-P. Raynaud, G. Koch, G. D. Chisholm, F. Di Silverio, P. Teillac, F. C. Da Silva, J. Cauquil, D. K. Chopin, F. C. Hamdy, M. Hanus, D. Hauri, A. Kalinteris, J. Marencak, A. Perier, and P. Perrin. Comparison of Phytotherapy (Permixon) with Finasteride in the Treatment of Benign Prostate Hyperplasia: A Randomized International Study of 1,098 Patients. *The Prostate,* 1996, 29, 231–240.

45. Champault, G., J. C. Patel, and A. M. Bonnard. A Double-blind Trial of an Extract of the Plant Serenoa repens in Benign Prostatic Hyperplasia. *British Journal of Clinical Pharmacology,* 1984, 18, 461–2.

46. Braeckman, J. The Extract of Serenoa repens in the Treatment of Benign Prostatic Hyperplasia: A Multicenter Open Study. *Current Therapeutic Research, Clinical and Experimental,* 1994, 55, 776–785.

47. Plosker, G. L. and R. N. Brogden. Serenoa repens (Permixon). A Review of Its

Pharmacology and Therapeutic Efficacy in Benign Prostatic Hyperplasia. *Drugs and Aging,* Nov. 1996, 9(5), 379–395.

48. Carraro, Raynaud, Koch, et al., op. cit.

49. Ibid.

50. Plosker and Brogden, op. cit.

51. Whitaker, J. *Dr. Whitaker's Guide to Natural Healing.* Rocklin, CA: Prima Publishing, 1995, p. 22.

52. Denis, L. J. Editorial Review of "Comparison of Phytotherapy (Permixon) with Finasteride in the Treatment of Benign Prostate Hyperplasia: A Randomized International Study of 1098 Patients. *The Prostate,* 1996, 29, 241–242.

53. Grasso, M., A. Montesano, A. Buonaguidi, M. Castelli, C. Lania, P. Rigatti, F. Rocco, B. M. Cesana, and C. Borghi. Comparative Effects of Alfuzosin Versus Serenoa repens in the Treatment of Symptomatic Benign Prostatic Hyperplasia. *Archives Espanoles de Urologia,* Jan. 1995, 48(1), 97–103.

54. Adriazola-Semino, M., J. L. Ortega-Lozano, E. Garcia-Cobo, E. Tejeda-Banez, and F. Romero-Rodriguez. Symptomatic Treatment of Benign Hypertrophy of the Prostate. Comparative Study of Prazosin and Serenoa repens. *Archives Espanoles de Urologia,* April 1992, 45(3), 211–213.

55. Ibid., p. 327.

56. Weiner and Weiner, op. cit., p. 291.

57. Steinman, D. Enlarged Prostate? Try Tree Bark. *Natural Health,* July/Aug. 1994, 24(4), 44, 46–47.

58. Barlet, A., J. Albrecht, A. Aubert, M. Fisher, F. Grof, H. G. Grothuesmann, J. C. Masson, E. Mazeman, R. Mermon, and H. Reichelt. Efficacy of Pygeum Africanum Extract in the Medical Therapy of Urination Disorders Due to Benign Prostatic Hyperplasia: Evaluation of Objective and Subjective Parameters. A Placebo-controlled Double-blind Multicenter Study. *Wiener Klinische Wochenschrift,* 23 Nov. 1990, 102(22), 667–673.

59. Steinman, op. cit.

60. Lichius, J. J., and C. Muth. The Inhibiting Effects of Urtica dioica Root Extracts on Experimentally Induced Prostatic Hyperplasia in the Mouse. *Planta Medica,* Aug. 1997, 63(4), 307–310.

61. Hirano, T., M. Homma, and K. Oka. Effects of Stinging Nettle Root Extracts and Their Steroidal Components on the Na+, K(+)-ATPase of the Benign Prostatic Hyperplasia. *Planta Medica,* Feb. 1994, 60(1), 30–33.

62. Cockett, A. T., Y. Aso, L. Denis, and S. Khoury. The International Prostate symptom Score (I-PSS) and Quality of Life Assessment. In *Proceedings of the International Consultation on Benign Prostatic Hyperplasia.* Paris, 1991, 280–281.

63. Klippel, K. F., D. M. Hiltl, and B. Schipp. A Multicentric, Placebo-controlled, Double-blind Clinical Trial of β-Sitosterol (Phytosterol) for the Treatment of Benign Prostatic Hyperplasia. *British Journal of Urology,* Sept. 1997, 80(3), 427–432.

64. Berges, R. R., J. Windeler, H. J. Trampisch, T. Senge, and the β-sitosterol Study Group. Randomized, Placebo-controlled, Double-blind Clinical Trial of β-sitosterol in Patients with Benign Prostatic Hyperplasia. *The Lancet,* 17 June 1995, 345(8964), 1529–1532.

65. Klippel, Hiltl, and Schipp, op. cit.

66. Berges, Windeler, Trampisch, et al., op. cit.

67. Tammela, op. cit., p. 359.

CHAPTER 4: THE MIRACLE OF CERNITIN

1. Most of the material for this chapter comes from Åke Asplund's autobiography *Searching the Source of Life and Vitality.* Singapore: Sanomin (SA) SDN.BHD., 1991.

2. Asplund, op. cit., p. 33.

3. *Grana Palynologica,* 1960, 2(2), 115–118.

4. Asplund, op. cit., p. 53–54.

5. Leander, G. A Preliminary Investigation on the Therapeutic Effect of Cernitin in Chronic Prostatovesiculitis. *Svenska Läkartidningen,* 1962, 59(45), 3296.

6. Ibid., p. 231.

7. Inada, T., T. Kitagawa, and M. Miyakawa. Use of Cernitin in Patients with Prostatic Hypertrophy. Undated manuscript distributed by Tobishi Pharmaceutical Co., Ltd., Tokyo, the distributor of Cernitin in Japan. At the time, the authors were all medical doctors affiliated with the Department of Urology at Kyoto University School of Medicine.

8. Takeuchi, H., Al Yamauchi, and T. Ueda, et al. Quantitative Evaluation on the Effectiveness of Cernitin on Benign Prostatic Hypertrophy. *Hinyokika Kiyo,* Feb. 1981, 27(2), 326–327.

9. Inada, Kitagawa, and Miyakawa, op. cit.

10. Kvanta, E. Sterols in Pollen. *Acta Chem. Scand.,* 1968, 22, 2161–2165.

11. Ohkoshi, M., N. Kawamura, and I. Nagakubo. Clinical Evaluation of Cernitin in Chronic Prostatitis. *Japanese Journal of Clinical Urology,* 1967, 21(1), 73–85.

12. Inada, Kitagawa, and Miyakawa, op. cit.

13. Maekawa, M., T. Kishimoto, R. Yasumoto, S. Wada, T. Harada, T. Ohara, E. Okajima, Y. Hirao, S. Ohzono, and K. Shimada. Clinical Evaluation of Cernitin on Benign Prostatic Hypertrophy—A Multiple Center Double-blind Study with Paraprost. *Hinyokika Kiyo,* April 1990, 36(4), 495–516.

14. Ebeling, op. cit.

15. Ibid., p. 155.

16. Bräuer, H., The Treatment of Benign Prostatic Hyperplasia with Phytopharmaca. A Comparative Study of Cernitin vs. Beta-sitosterol. *Therapiewoche,* 1986, 36, 1686–1696.

17. Becker, H., and L. Ebeling. Conservative Treatment of Benign Prostatic Hyperplasia (BPH) with Cernitin N. *Urologe B,* 1988, 28, 301–306.

18. Becker, H., and L. Ebeling. Phytotherapy of BPH with Cernitin N. Results of a Controlled Clinical Study. *Urologe B,* 1991, 31, 113–116.

19. Buck, A. C., R. Cox, R. W. Rees, L. Ebeling, and A. John. Treatment of Outflow Tract Obstruction due to Benign Prostatic Hyperplasia with the Pollen Extract, Cernitin. A Double-blind, Placebo-controlled Study. *British Journal of Urology,* 1990(Oct.), 66(4), 398–404.

20. Rugendorff, E. W., W. Weidner, L. Ebeling, A. C. Buck. Results of Treatment with Pollen Extract (Cernitin N) in Chronic Prostatitis and Prostatodynia. *British Journal of Urology,* April 1993, 71(4), 433–438.

21. Buck, A. C., R. W. Rees, L. Ebeling. Treatment of Chronic Prostatitis and Prostatodynia with Pollen Extract. *British Journal of Urology,* Nov. 1989, 64(5), 496–499.

22. Yasumoto, R., H. Kawanishi, T. Tsujino, M. Tsujita, N. Nishisaki, A. Horii, and T. Kishimoto. Clinical Evaluation of Long-term Treatment Using Cernitin Pollen Extract in Patients with Benign Prostatic Hyperplasia. *Clinical Therapeutics,* Jan. 1995, 17(1), 82–87.

23. Dutkiewicz, S. Usefulness of Cernitin in the Treatment of Benign Prostatic Hyperplasia. *International Urology and Nephrology,* 1996, 28(1), 49–53.

24. Habib, F. K., M. Ross, A. C. Buck, L. Ebeling, and A. Lewenstein. In Vitro Evaluation of the Pollen Extract, Cernitin T-60, in the Regulation of Prostate Cell Growth. *British Journal of Urology,* Oct. 1990, 66(4), 393–397.

25. Zhang, H., F. K. Habib, M. Ross, U. Burger, A. Lewenstein, K. Rose, and J. C. Jaton. Isolation and Characterization of a Cyclic Hydroxamic Acid from a Pollen Extract, Which Inhibits Cancerous Cell Growth in Vitro. *Journal of Medicinal Chemistry,* 17 Feb. 1995, 38(4), 735–738.

26. Habib, F. K., M. Ross, A. Lewenstein, X. Zhang, and J. C. Jaton. Identification of a Prostate Inhibitory Substance in a Pollen Extract. *The Prostate,* March 1995, 26(3), 133–139.

27. Salmon, J. W. "Introduction." In *Alternative Medicines, Popular and Policy Perspectives,* J. W. Salmon, ed. NY: Tavistock Publications, 1984, p. 6.

28. American Medical Association. *Reader's Guide to Alternative Health Methods.* Milwaukee, WI, American Medical Association, 1993.

29. American Medical Association, op. cit., p. 69.

30. Morton, M., and M. Morton. *Five Steps to Selecting the Best Alternative Medicine.* NY: New World Library, 1997.

31. Salmon, op. cit., p. 9.

32. Taylor, R. C. R. "Alternative Medicine and the Medical Encounter in Britain and the United States." In Salmon, op. cit., pp. 191–228.

33. Wallis, R., and P. Morley. "Introduction." In R. Wallis and P. Morley, eds. *Marginal Medicine.* London: Peter Owen, 1976,

34. Salmon, J. W., and H. S. Berliner. Health Policy Implications of the Holistic Health Movement. *Journal of Health Politics, Policy and Law,* 1980, 5(3), 535–553.

CHAPTER 5: THE PROSTATE CURE: A SEVEN-STEP PROACTIVE PROGRAM

1. Galland, L. How to Be Healthy. Conclusions from Dr. Leo Galland's 30 Years of Research. *Bottom Line Personal,* 15 Dec. 1997, 11–12.

2. Rous, op. cit., p. 186.

3. Ibid., p. 183.

4. Fawzy, A., C. Fontenot, R. Guthrie, and M. M. Baudier. Practice Patterns Among Primary Care Physicians in Benign Prostatic Hyperplasia and Prostate Cancer. *Family Medicine,* May 1997, 29(5), 321–325.

5. Walsh and Worthington, op. cit., p. 95.

6. Fiore, N. Living Well with Cancer. *Bottom Line Health,* December 1997, 13.

7. Rippe, J. How to Start Your Own Walking Program. *Bottom Line Health,* Nov. 1997, 8–9.

8. *Unpublicized Health Breakthroughs, Warnings & Secrets,* NY: Boardroom, Inc., 1997, p. 15.

9. Evans, W. J. Biomarkers. The Keys to Lifelong Vitality. *Bottom Line Tomorrow,* Nov. 1997, 5(11), 1–2.

10. Rippe, op. cit.

11. Aerobic Exercise. *Harvard Women's Health Watch,* Nov. 1997, 5(3), 6.

12. Ibid.

13. Binney, R., ed. *The Complete Manual of Fitness and Well-Being.* NY: Viking Penguin, Inc., 1984, p. 100.

14. Ibid.

15. Rippe, op. cit.

16. Salmans, op. cit., p. 88.

17. Evans, W. J. Biomarkers. The Keys to Lifelong Vitality. *Bottom Line Tomorrow,* Nov. 1997, 5(11), 1–3.

18. Salmans, op. cit., p. 88.

19. Gu, F. Changes in the Prevalence of Benign Prostatic Hyperplasia in China. *Chinese Medical Journal* (English), 1997, 110 (3), 163–166.

20. Carlson, R. *Don't Sweat the Small Stuff . . . and It's All Small Stuff.* New York: Hyperion, 1997.

21. Smith, C. A., and L. W. Morris. Effects of Stimulative and Sedative Music on Cognitive and Emotional Components of Anxiety. *Psychological Reports,* 1976, 38, 1187–1193.

22. Courtright, P., S. Johnson, M. A. Baumgartner, M. Jordan, and J. C. Webster. Dinner Music: Does It Affect the Behavior of Psychiatric Inpatients? *Journal of Psychosocial Nursing,* 1990, 28(3), 37–40.

23. For information on Steven Halpern's music, contact his company at P.O. Box 2644, San Anselmo, CA 94979-2644, tel. (800) 909-0707. His e-mail address is innerpeacemusic@innerpeacemusic; and his website can be reached at www.steven.stevenhalpern.com.

24. Sobel, D. S., and R. Ornstein. Imagery: How to Use Your Imagination to Improve Your Health. *Mind/Body Health Newsletter,* 1997, 6(3), 3–6.

25. Beck, A. T. *Love Is Never Enough.* NY: Harper & Row, 1988.

26. Burns, D. D. *Feeling Good.* NY: William Morrow & Co., Inc., 1980.

27. Fiore, N. *The Road Back to Health: Coping with the Emotional Aspects of Cancer.* Berkeley, CA: Celestial Arts, 1995.

28. Published in paperback in 1997 by Hyperion, New York.

29. Carlson, R. *Don't Sweat the Small Stuff . . . and It's All Small Stuff.* NY: Hyperion, 1997, p. 7.

30. Ibid., pp. 81–83.

31. Cohen, M. Caring for Ourselves Can Be Funny Business. *Holistic Nursing Practice,* 1990, 4(4), 1–11.

32. Tennant, K. F. Laugh It Off. The Effect of Humor on the Well-Being of the Older Adult. *Journal of Gerontological Nursing,* 1 Dec. 1990, 16(12), 11–17.

33. Fry, Jr., W. F. The Physiological Effects of Humor, Mirth, and Laughter. *JAMA,* 1 April 1992, 267(13), 1857–1858.

34. Hudak, D. A., J. A. Dale, M. A. Hudak, and D. E. DeGood. Effects of Humorous Stimuli and Sense of Humor on Discomfort. *Psychological Reports,* Dec. 1991, 69(3), 779–786.

35. Danzer, A., J. A. Dale, and H. L. Klions. Effect of Exposure to Humorous Stimuli on Induced Depression. *Psychological Reports,* June 1990, 66 (3 pt. 1), 1027–1036.

36. Dugan, D. O. Laughter and Tears: Best Medicine for Stress. *Nursing Forum,* Jan. 1989, XXIV(1), 18–26.

37. Erdman, L. Laughter Therapy for Patients with Cancer. *Oncology Nursing Forum,* 1991, 18(8), 1359–1363.

38. Davidhizar, R., and M. Bowen. The Dynamics of Laughter. *Archives of Psychiatric Nursing,* April 1992, 6(2), 132–137.

39. Henry, B. M., and L. E. Moody. Energize with Laughter. *Nursing Success Today,* 1 Jan. 1985, 2(1), 5–8, 36.

40. Dugan, op. cit.

41. Fry, op. cit.

42. Ibid.

43. Fry, Jr., W. J. "Humor and the Human Cardiovascular System." In *The Study of Humor,* H. Mindess and J. Turek, eds. Los Angeles: Antioch University, 1979.

44. Dugan, op. cit.

45. Labott, S. M., S. Ahleman, M. E. Wolever, and R. B. Martin. The Physiological and Psychological Effects of the Expression and Inhibition of Emotion. *Behavioral Medicine,* 1990, 16(4), 182–189.

46. Published in New York by W. W. Norton, 1979.

47. Tennant, K. F. Laugh It Off. The Effect of Humor on the Well-Being of the Older Adult. *Journal of Gerontological Nursing,* 1 Dec. 1990, 16(12), 11–17.

48. We discovered this wonderful and appropriate pun in the writing of Goodman, J. B. Laughing Matters: Taking Your Job Seriously and Yourself Lightly. *JAMA,* 1 April 1992, 267(11), 1858.

49. Sullivan, D. Humor and Health. *Journal of Gerontological Nursing,* 1988, 14(1), 20–24.

50. Contact them at 222 S. Meramec, Suite #303, St. Louis, MO, tel. (314) 863-6232. Their website address is http://www.ideanurse.com/aath/.

CHAPTER 6: LIVING WELL IS THE BEST REVENGE

1. Cousins, op. cit.

2. McCall, T., B. Healy, and W. Castelli. Secrets of Good Health for Men and Women in Their 40s, Their 50s, and 60+. *Bottom Line Personal,* 1 Nov. 1997, 18(21), pp. 9–10.

3. Salmans, op. cit., pp. 84–85.

4. Walsh and Worthington. op. cit., p. 29.

5. Shibata and Whittemore. op. cit.

6. Berman, B. M., and D. B. Larson, eds. *Alternative Medicine: Expanding Medical Horizons. A Report to the National Institute of Health on Alternative Medical Systems and Practices in the United States.* Washington, D.C.: U.S. Government Printing Office, 1994.

7. Oishi, K., K. Okada, O. Yoshida, H. Yamabe, Y. Ohno, R. B. Hayes, and F. H. Schroeder. A Case-control Study of Prostatic Cancer with Reference to Dietary Habits. *Prostate,* 1988, 12(2), 179–190.

8. Shintani, T. T., C. K. Hughes, S. Bechlam, and H. K. O'Connor. Obesity and Cardiovascular Risk Intervention Through the Ad Libitum Feeding of a Traditional Hawaiian Diet. *American Journal of Clinical Nutrition,* 1991, 53, 1647s–1651s.

9. Morgan, op. cit., p. 272.

10. Salmans, op. cit., p. 84. See also Walsh and Worthington. op. cit., p. 30.

11. Jaroff, op. cit., p. 65.

12. Rosenfeld, I. The Food Superstars. Best Sources of Disease-Fighting Phytochemicals. *Bottom Line Health,* Nov. 1997, p. 15.

13. Clinton, S. K., and W. J. Visek. Wheat Bran and the Induction of Intestinal Benzo(a)pyrene Hydroxylase by Dietary Benszo(a)pyrene. *Journal of Nutrition,* 1989, 119(3), 395–402.

14. Rosenfeld, op. cit., p. 82.

15. Ibid., p. 82.

16. Ibid., p. 83.

17. Walford, R. L. Calorie Restriction. The Aggressive Anti-Aging Plan. *Bottom Line Health,* Feb. 1998, 12(2), 13–14.

18. Willett, W. C., B. F. Polk, J. S. Morris, M. J. Stampfer, S. Pressel, B. Rosner, J. O. Taylor, K. Schneider, and C. G. Hames. Prediagnostic Serum Selenium and Risk of Cancer. *The Lancet* 16 July 1983, 2(8342), 130–134.

19. Clark, L. C., G. F. Combs, Jr., B. W. Burnbull, E. H. Slate, D. K. Chalker, J. Chow, L. S. Davis, R. A. Glover, G. F. Graham, E. G. Gross, A. Krongrad, J. L. Lesher, Jr., H. K. Park, B. B. Sanders, Jr., C. L. Smith, J. R. Taylor, and the Nutritional Prevention of Cancer Study Group. Effects of Selenium Supplementation for Cancer Prevention in Patients with Carcinoma of the Skin. A Randomized Controlled Trial. *JAMA,* 25 Dec. 1996, 276(24), 1957–1963.

20. Habib, Hammond, Lee, et al. op. cit.

21. Mindell, op. cit., p. 266.

22. Taylor, N. *Green Tea.* N.Y.: Kensington Publishing Corp., 1998, p. 114.

23. Can Green Tea Help Prevent Cancer? *University of California at Berkeley Wellness Letter.* Dec. 1997, 14(3), 1–2.

24. Taylor, op. cit., p. 2.

25. *Bottom Line Personal,* 1 Nov. 1997, 18(21), p. 3.

26. Fujiki, H., S. Yoshizawa, T. Horiuchi, M. Suganumu, J. Yatsumani, S. Nishiwaki, S. Okabe, R. Nishiwaki-Matsushima, T. Okuda, and T. Sugimura. Anticarcinogenic Effects of (–)-epigallocatechin Gallate. *Preventive Medicine,* July 1992, 21(4), 503–509.

27. Study cited in Taylor, op. cit., with original reference given as Oguni, I, S. J. Cheng, P. Z. Lin, and U. Hara. Protection Against Cancer Risk by Japanese Green Tea. *Preventive Medicine,* 1992, 21, 332.

28. Taylor, op. cit., p. 40 cites a study taken from the Internet 11/27/96 by Carlin, B. I., T. G. Pretlow, T. P. Pretlow, H. Mukhtar, R. R. Mohan, R. Agrawal, and M. I. Resnick, entitled "Green Tea Polyphenols Inhibit Growth of Prostate Cancer Zenograft CWR-22 and Decrease Ornithine Decarboxylase Activity: Implications for Prostate Cancer Chemoprevention."

29. Taylor, op. cit.

30. Ibid.

31. Walsh and Worthington. op. cit., p. 29.

32. Morgan, op. cit., p. 274.

33. Rosso, J., and S. Lukins. *The New Basics Cookbook.* NY: Workman Publishing.

34. Araki, H., H. Watanabe, T. Mishina, and M. Nakao. High-risk Group for Benign Prostatic Hypertrophy. *Prostate,* 1983, 4(3), 253–264.

35. Walsh and Worthington. op. cit., p. 29–30.

36. Herbert, V. America's Very Dangerous Vitamin Craze. *Bottom Line Health,* Jan. 1998, 12,(1), 1–3.

37. Diet and Cancer. *Bottom Line Health,* Jan. 1988, 12(1), 9–12.

38. Rosenfeld, op. cit.

39. Tomatoes and Heart Attack. *Bottom Line Personal,* 1 Jan. 1998, 19(1), p. 1.

40. Weiner, M. A., and J. A. Weiner. *Herbs that Heal.* Mill Valley, CA: Quantum Books, 1994, p. 159.

41. Ibid., p. 160.

42. Ibid., p. 161.

43. Diet and Cancer. op. cit.

44. Clinton and Visek, op. cit.

45. Margolis and Carter. op. cit., p. 25.

46. Walsh and Worthington. op. cit., p. 33.

47. Margolis and Carter. op. cit., p. 25.

48. Thomas, M. K., D. M. Lloyd-Jones, R. I. Thadhani, A. C. Shaw, D. J. Deraska, B. T. Kitch, E. C. Vamvakas, I. M. Dick, R. L. Prince, and J. S. Finkelstein. Hypovitaminosis D in Medical Inpatients. *New England Journal of Medicine,* 19 March 1988, 338(12), 777–783.

49. Don't Overlook Vitamin D for Osteoporosis Prevention. *Environmental Nutrition,* May 1998, 21(5), 8.

50. Herbert, op. cit.

51. Moul, op. cit.

52. Liehr, J. G. Vitamin C Reduces the Incidence and Severity of Renal Tumors Induced by Estradiol and Diethylstilbestrol. *American Journal of Clinical Nutrition,* 1991, 54, 1256S–1260S.

53. Pauling, L. Effect of Ascorbic Acid on Incidence of Spontaneous Mammary Tumors and UV-light Induced Skin Tumors in Mice. *American Journal of Clinical Nutrition,* 1991, 54, 1252S–1255S.

54. Cameron, E., L. Pauling, and B. Leibovitz. Ascorbic Acid and Cancer: A Review. *Cancer Research,* 1979, 39, 663–681.

55. Block, G. Vitamin C Status and Cancer. Epidemiologic Evidence of Reduced Risk. *Annals of the New York Academy of Science,* 1992, 669, 280–292.

56. Maramag, C., M. Menon, K. C. Balaji, P. G. Reddy, and S. Laxmanan. Effect of Vitamin C on Prostate Cancer Cells In Vitro: Effect on Cell Number, Viability, and DNA Synthesis. *The Prostate,* 1997, 32, 188–195.

57. Herbert, op. cit.

58. The Alpha-tocopherol, Beta-carotene Cancer Prevention Study Group: The Effect of Vitamin E and Beta-carotene on the Incidence of Lung Cancer and Other Cancers in Male Smokers. *New England Journal of Medicine,* 1994, 330, 1029–1035.

59. Stampfer, M. J., C. H. Hennekins, J. E. Manson. Vitamin E consumption and the risk of coronary disease in women. *New England Journal of Medicine,* 328: 1444–1449, 1993.

60. Rimm E. B., M. J. Stampfer, A. Ascherio. Vitamin E consumption and the risk of coronary heart disease in men. *New England Journal of Medicine,* 328:1450–1456, 1993.

61. Herbert, op. cit.

62. Whelan, P., B. E. Walker, and J. Kelleher. Zinc, Vitamin A, and Prostatic Cancer. *British Journal of Urology,* Oct. 1983, 55(5), 525–528.

63. Salmans, op. cit., p. 37.

64. Werbach, M. *Healing with Food.* NY: HarperPerennial, 1993, p. 332.

65. Ibid.

66. Fahim, M. S., M. Wang, M. F. Sutcu, and Z. Fahim. Zinc Arginine, a 5 Alpha-reductase Inhibitor, Reduces Rat Ventral Prostate Weight and DNA without Affecting Testicular Function. *Andrologia,* Nov. 1993, 25(6), 369–375.

67. Habib, F. K., G. L. Hammond, I. R. Lee, J. B. Dawson, M. K. Mason, P. H. Smith, and S. R. Stitch. Metal-androgen Interrelationships in Carcinoma and Hyperplasia of the Human Prostate. *Journal of Endocrinology,* Oct. 1976, 71(1), 133–141.

68. Whelan, P., B. E. Walker, and J. Kelleher. op. cit.

69. Hurley, B. *The Good Herb.* NY: William Morrow and Company, Inc., 1995, p. 380.

70. Judd, A. M., R. M. Macleod, and I. W. Login. Zinc Acutely, Selectively and Reversibly Inhibits Pituitary Prolactin Secretion. *Brain Research,* 27 Feb. 1984, 294(1), 190–192.

71. Leake, A., G. D. Chisholm, and F. K. Habib. The Effect of Zinc on the 5 Alpha-reduction of Testosterone by the Hyperplastic Human Prostate Gland. *Journal of Steroid Biochemistry and Molecular Biology,* Feb. 1984, 20(2), 651–655.

72. Salmans, op. cit., p. 38.

73. Evans, G. W., and E. C. Johnson. Effect of Iron, Vitamin B-6 and Picolinic Acid on Zinc Absorption in the Rat. *Journal of Nutrition,* Jan. 1981, 111(1), 68–75.

74. Charles, R. *Food for Healing.* London: Mandarin Paperbacks, 1995, p. 127.

75. Haas, E. M. Staying Healthy with Nutrition. Report on Zinc from the Internet's Health World Online (http://www.healthy.net/library/books/Haas/minerals/zn.htm).

76. Herbs and Medicines May Not Mix. *Bottom Line Personal,* 1 Jan. 1998, 19(1), p. 16.

77. Winter, A., and R. Winter. *Eat Right, Be Bright.* NY: St. Martins Press, 1988.

78. Graedon, J., and T. Graedon. *Graedons' Best Medicine: From Herbal Remedies to High-Tech Rx Breakthroughs.* NY: Bantam Books, 1991, p. 329.

79. Kupeli, B., T. Soygur, K. Aydos, E. Ozdiler, and S. Kupeli. The Role of Cigarette Smoking in Prostatic Enlargement. *British Journal of Urology,* Aug. 1997, 80(2), 201–204.

80. Lumey, L. H., B. Pittman, E. A. Zang, and E. L. Wynder. Cigarette Smoking and Prostate Cancer: No Relation with Six Measures of Lifetime Smoking Habits in a Large Case-Control Study Among U.S. Whites. *The Prostate,* 1997, 33, 195–200.

CHAPTER 7: PROSTATE CANCER

1. Margolis and Carter, op. cit., p. 23.

2. Culkin, D. J., and A. H. Agha. Localized Prostate Cancer: An Update. *Hospital Medicine,* 1997, 35(5), 25–26, 29–36, 45.

3. Culkin and Agha, op. cit.

4. Mettlin, C. Changes in Patterns of Prostate Cancer Care in the United States: Results of American College of Surgeons Commission on Cancer Studies, 1974–1993. *The Prostate,* 1997, 32, 221–226.

5. Schmidt, J. D. The Case for Early Endocrine Treatment of Advanced or Metastatic Prostate Cancer. *The Prostate,* 1996, 28, 201–204.

6. Mettlin, op. cit.

7. Schmid, H. P., J. E. McNeal, and T. A. Stamey. Observations on the Doubling Time of Prostate Cancer. The Use of Serial Prostate-specific Antigen in Patients with Untreated Disease as a Measure of Increasing Cancer Volume. *Cancer,* 1993, 71, 2031–2040.

8. Culkin and Agha, op. cit.

9. Jaroff, op. cit.

10. Margolis and Carter, op. cit., p. 24.

11. Walsh and Worthington, op. cit., p. 29.

12. Morgan, B. L. G. *Nutrition Prescription.* NY: Crown Publishers, Inc., p. 270.

13. Culkin and Agha, op. cit.

14. Emmons, S. "Going Public." *Los Angeles Times,* 19 March 1997, pp. E-1, E-6.

15. Margolis and Carter, op. cit., p. 24.

16. Ibid.

17. Shibata, A., and A. C. Whittemore. Genetic Predisposition to Prostate Cancer: Possible Explanations for Ethnic Differences in Risk. *The Prostate,* 1997, 32, 65–72.

18. Walsh and Worthington, op. cit., p. 27.

19. Jaroff, op. cit., p. 65.

20. Culkin and Agha, op. cit.

21. Thompson, I. M., C. A. Coltman, Jr., and J. Crowley. Chemoprevention of Prostate Cancer: The Prostate Cancer Prevention Trial. *The Prostate,* 1997, 33, 217–221.

22. Walsh and Worthington, op. cit., p. 30.

23. Margolis and Carter, op. cit., p. 25.

24. Shibata and Whittemore, op. cit.

25. Margolis and Carter, op. cit., p. 25.

26. Walsh and Worthington, op. cit., p. 30.

27. Schwartz, G. C., and C. L. Hanchette. Geographic Patterns of Prostate Cancer Mortality. *Cancer,* 1992, 70, 2865.

28. Emmons, op. cit.

29. Catalona, W. J. Clinical Utility of Measurements of Free and Total Prostate-Specific Antigen (PSA): A Review. *The Prostate Supplement,* 1996, 7, 64–69.

30. Walsh and Worthington, op. cit., p. 42.

31. Coley, C. M., M. J. Barry, C. Fleming, et al. Early Detection of Prostate Cancer, Part I; op. cit. Part II: Estimating the risks, Benefits, and Costs. *Annals of*

Internal Medicine, 1 March 1997, 126(5), 468–47. Coley, C. M., M. J. Barry, and A. G. Mulley for the College of Physicians. Screening for Prostate Cancer. *Annals of Internal Medicine,* 1 March 1997, 126(5), 480–484.

32. Middleton, R. G. Prostate Cancer: Are We Screening and Treating Too Much? *Annals of Internal Medicine,* 1 March 1997, 126(5), 465–467.

33. Jaroff, op. cit., pp. 58–59.

34. Walsh and Worthington, op. cit., p. 41.

35. Culkin and Agha, op. cit.

36. Coley, C. M., M. J. Barry, C. Fleming, and A. G. Mulley. Early Detection of Prostate Cancer. Part I: Prior Probability and Effectiveness of Tests. The American College of Physicians. *Annals of Internal Medicine,* 1 March 1997, 126(5), 394–406.

37. Salmans, op. cit., p. 72.

38. Ravery, V., and Boccon-Gibod, L. Free/Total Prostate-Specific Antigen Ratio— Hope and Controversies. *European Urology,* 1997, 31, 385–388.

39. Ibid.

40. Catalona, W. J. Clinical Utility of Measurements of Free and Total Prostate-Specific Antigen (PSA): A Review. *The Prostate Supplement,* 1996, 7, 64–69.

41. Vetrosky, D. T., L. Gerdom, G. L. White, Jr. Prostate Cancer—Pathology, Diagnosis, and Management. *Clinician Reviews,* 1997, 7(5), 79–81, 85–86, 89–91, 94–96, 99–100.

42. van Iersel, M. P., W. P. J. Witjes, C. M. G. Thomas, M. F. G. Segers, G. O. N. Oosterhof, and F. M. J. Debruyne. Review on the Simultaneous Determination of Total Prostate-Specific Antigen and Free Prostate-Specific Antigen. *The Prostate Supplement,* 1996, 7, 48–57.

43. Walsh and Worthington, op. cit., p. 45.

44. Etzioni, R., Y. Shen, J. C. Petteway, and M. K. Brawer. Age-Specific Prostate-Specific Antigen: A Reassessment. *The Prostate Supplement,* 1996, 7, 70–77.

45. Wolff, J. M., H. Borchers, W. Boeckmann, F. K. Habib, and G. Jakse. Improved Discrimination Between Prostatic Carcinoma and Benign Prostatic Hyperplasia by Determination of Free Prostate-specific Antigen Percentage. *Urologe A,* May 1997, 36(3), 255–258. This article is in German. For an American version, see Wolff, J. M., W. Boeckmann, J. Effert, F. K. Habib, and G. Jakse. Increased Discrimination Between Benign Prostatic Hyperplasia and Prostate Cancer Through

Measurement of Percentage Free PSA. *Anticancer Research,* July 1997, 17(4B), 2993–2994.

46. Gilson, G., S. Lamy, and R. L. Humbel. First Clinical Results with Enzymun-Test for Free PSA. *Anticancer Research,* July 1997, 17(4B), 2861–2864.

47. van Iersel, Witjes, Thomas, et al., op. cit.

48. de la Taille, A., A. Houlgatte, P. Houdeletter, P. Berlizot, J. Ramirez, and I. Ricordel. Value of Free/Total Prostate Specific Antigen in the Early Diagnosis of Prostate Cancer. *Progres en Urologie,* April 1997, 7(2), 240–245.

49. Filella, X., J. Alcover, R. Molina, A. Rodreguez, P. Carretero, and A. M. Ballesta. Clinical Evaluation of Free PSA/Total PSA (Prostate-Specific Antigen) Ratio in the Diagnosis of Prostate Cancer. *European Journal of Cancer,* July 1997, 33(8), 1226–1229.

50. van Iersel, Witjes, Thomas, et al., op. cit.

51. Vashi, A. R., and J. E. Oesterling. Percent Free Prostate-specific Antigen: Entering a New Era in the Detection of Prostate Cancer. *Mayo Clinic Proceedings,* April 1997, 72(4), 337–344.

52. Chen, Z., H. Chen, and T. A. Stamey. Prostate Specific Antigen in Benign Prostatic Hyperplasia: Purification and Characterization. *Journal of Urology,* June 1997, 157(6), 2166–2170.

53. Oesterling, J. E., S. J. Jacobsen, C. G. Chute, H. A. Guess, C. J. Girman, L. A. Panser, and M. M. Lieber. Serum PSA in a Community-based Population of Healthy Men. *JAMA,* 1993, 270, 860–864.

54. Catalona, op. cit.

55. Etzioni, Shen, Petteway, and Brawer, op. cit.

56. Salmans, op. cit., p. 76.

57. Vetrosky, Gerdom, and White, op. cit.

58. Walsh and Worthington, op. cit., p. 51.

59. Margolis and Carter, op. cit., p. 27.

60. Garnick, M. B. *The Patient's Guide to Prostate Cancer.* NY: Plume, 1996, p. 21.

61. Salcedo, op. cit., p. 65.

62. Vetrosky, Gerdom, and White, op. cit.

63. Culkin and Agha. op. cit.

64. Salmans, op. cit., p. 81.

65. Salcedo, op. cit., p. 69.

66. Mettlin, op. cit.

67. Smith, P. H. Carcinoma of Prostate: Case Against Immediate Hormonal Therapy. *The Prostate,* 1996, 28, 205–208.

68. Walsh and Worthington, op. cit., p. 262.

69. Jaroff, op. cit., p. 62.

70. Leland, J. A Pill for Impotence? *Newsweek,* 17 Nov. 1997, pp. 62–67.

71. Jaroff, op. cit., p. 62.

72. Gorman, C. The Politics of Bob Dole's Prostate Cancer. *Time,* 1 April 1996, 147(14), p. 63.

73. Jaroff, op. cit., p. 63.

74. Schmid, H. P., J. E. McNeal, and T. A. Stamey. Observations on the Doubling Time of Prostate Cancer. The Use of Serial Prostate-specific Antigen in Patients with Untreated Disease as a Measure of Increasing Cancer Volume. *Cancer,* 1993, 71, 2031–2040.

75. Friedman, R. M., ed. PSA—An Imperfect Test. *University of California at Berkeley Wellness Letter,* Nov. 1997, 14(2), p. 6.

76. Ibid.

77. Smith, op. cit.

78. Mettlin, op. cit.

79. Walsh, P. C., A. W. Partin, and J. I. Epstein. Cancer Control and Quality of Life Following Anatomical Radical Retropubic Prostatectomy: Results at 10 Years. *Journal of Urology,* 1994, 152, 1831–1836.

80. Mettlin, op. cit.

81. Jaroff, op. cit., p. 62.

82. Thiel, R., and R. Ackermann. Avoiding Complications of Radical Retropubic Prostatectomy. *European Urology,* 1997, 3 (suppl. 3) 9–15.

83. Korda, op. cit.

84. Ibid.

85. Shir, Y., S. N. Raja, S. M. Frank, and C. B. Brendler. Intraoperative Blood Loss During Radical Retropubic Prostatectomy: Epidural versus General Anesthesia. *Urology,* 1995, 45, 993–999.

86. Oefelein, M. G., L. A. Colangelo, A. W. Rademaker, and K. T. McVary. Intraoperative Blood Loss and Prognosis in Prostate Cancer Patients Undergoing Radical Retropubic Prostatectomy. *Journal of Urology,* 1995, 154, 442–447.

87. Salcedo, op. cit., p. 98.

88. Stamey, T. A., M. K. Gerrari, and H. P. Schmid. The Value of Serial Prostate Specific Antigen Determinations 5 Years after Radiotherapy; Steeply Increasing Values Characterize 80% of Patients. *Journal of Urology,* 1993, 150, 1856–1859.

89. Onik, G. M., J. K. Cohen, G. D. Reyes, B. Rubinsky, Z. Chang, and J. Baust. Transrectal Ultrasound-Guided Percutaneous Radical Cryosurgical Ablation of the Prostate. *Cancer,* 15 Aug. 1993, 72(4), 1291–1299.

90. Schachter, M. Alternative Approaches to Prostate Cancer. An article printed on the Health World Online at http://www.healthy.net.library/articles/Schacter/prostate.d.htm.

91. Rous, op. cit., p. 226.

92. Ibid.

93. Fosså, S. D., H. Wæhre, K.-H. Kurth, J. Hetherington, H. Bakke, D. A. Rustad, and Remi Skånvik. Influence of Urological Morbidity on Quality of Life in Patients with Prostate Cancer. *European Urology,* 1997, 3 (suppl. 3), 3–8.

94. Margolis and Carter, op. cit., p. 35.

95. Onik, Cohen, and Reyes, op. cit.

96. Emmons, op. cit.

97. This information comes from a paper by T. A. Stamey, M.D., (professor at Stanford University School of Medicine), "Prostate Cancer: Who Should Be Treated?" and presented on the OncoLink website of the University of Pennsylvania Cancer Center at http://oncolink.upenn.edu/disease/prostate/treatment/stamey.html.

98. Schachter, op. cit.

99. Bolla, M., D. Gonzalez, P. Warde, J. B. Dubois, R. O. Mirimanoff, G. Storme, J. Bernier, A. Kuten, C. Sternberg, T. Gil, L. Collette, and M. Pierart. Improved Survival in Patients with Locally Advanced Prostate Cancer Treated with Radiotherapy and Goserelin. *New England Journal of Medicine,* 31 July 1997, 337(5), 295–300.

100. *Unpublicized Health Breakthroughs, Warnings & Secrets.* NY: Boardroom Inc., 1997, p. 18.

101. Schmidt, op. cit.

102. This information was received over the Internet from The Prostate Cancer Info Link at http://comed.com/Prostate/Faqs.html.

103. Fosså, Wæhre, Kurth, et al., op. cit.

104. Korda, op. cit., p. 254.

CHAPTER 8: CONCLUSION

1. Randrup, E. R., and N. Baum. Pharmacologic Management of Benign Prostatic Hyperplasia. *Hospital Medicine,* 1997, 33(11), 43–44, 47–50, 53.

2. Nixon, P. New Clinical Trial of Medical Therapy for Benign Prostatic Hyperplasia. *Drug Benefits Trends,* 1997, 9(3), 44–45.

3. Keetch, op. cit.

4. Singer, A. J., and A. Starr. Outpatient Transurethral Resection of the Prostate. *Infections in Urology,* 1995, 8(2), 37–38.

A P P E N D I X

AMERICAN UROLOGICAL ASSOCIATION (AUA)
SYMPTOM SCORE

The following questionnaire* was developed by the AUA to help men evaluate the severity of their lower urinary tract symptoms from BPH. It is used by individual men and by research groups to determine not only severity but success of treatment by diminishing symptoms. Circle the one number on each line that correctly describes your symptoms.

* Adapted from Barry, M. J., F. J. Fowler, Jr., M. P. O'Leary, R. C. Bruskewitz, H. L. Holtgrewe, W. K. Mebust, and A. T. Cockett. The American Urological Association Symptom Index for Benign Prostatic Hyperplasia. The Measurement Committee of the American Urological Association. *Journal of Urology,* 1992, 148, 1549–1557.

Over the past month how often ...	Not at all	Less than 1 time in 5	Less than half the time	About half the time	More than half the time	Almost always
Have you had the sensation of not emptying your bladder completely after you have finished urinating? (Incomplete emptying)	0	1	2	3	4	5
Have you had to urinate again less than two hours after you finished urinating? (Frequency)	0	1	2	3	4	5
Have you found you stopped and started again several times when you urinated? (Intermittency)	0	1	2	3	4	5
Have you found it difficult to postpone urination? (Urgency)	0	1	2	3	4	5
Have you had a weak urinary stream? (Weak stream)	0	1	2	3	4	5
Have you had to push or strain to begin urination? (Straining)	0	1	2	3	4	5
How many times did you most typically get up to urinate from the time you went to bed at night until the time you got up in the morning? (Nocturia)	0	1	2	3	4	5

Scores of 0 to 7 represent mild symptoms; 8 to 19 suggests moderate symptoms. A score of 20 to 35 indicates severe symptoms.

GLOSSARY

ablation When used in the case of prostate cancer, it means destroying cancer cells.

acid phosphatase An enzyme made by both normal and malignant cells in the prostate. If malignant cells break out of the prostate and move to other places in the body, they nevertheless continue to make acid phosphatase, thus elevating its value above the normal level in a blood test. Therefore, elevated blood serum levels of acid phosphatase indicate that prostatic cancer cells have spread outside the prostate gland. It cannot be used as a screening test to detect early prostatic cancer still confined within the gland itself.

acute A disorder or infection in the body that reaches a crisis rapidly rather than with a slow, progressive onset.

acute bacterial prostatitis A form of prostatitis associated with urinary tract infections, the presence of bacteria in urinary cultures, and an abundance of white blood cells in prostatic secretions. Its onset is sudden rather than by slow growth of prostatic tissue as in BPH.

adenocarcinoma The most common type of prostate tumor, and the type most responsive to hormonal therapy. It develops in glandular tissue (specifically the acinar glands) located in the posterior peripheral zone of the prostate.

age-specific or age-adjusted reference range of PSA   The normal values of PSA modified or correlated to the age of the patient in order to more accurately determine the significance of PSA numbers.

alpha-adrenergic blockers   Medications that act on the bladder neck and the prostate by relaxing their smooth muscle tissue, thereby relieving the pressure on the urethral channel and opening the passage to increase urine flow.

anatomic prostatectomy   *See* **nerve-sparing prostatectomy.**

androgens   All the male hormones, which are necessary for the development and functioning of male sexual organs and male characteristics (facial hair, deep voice). More often, the term is used as a general reference to testosterone and dihydrotestosterone (*see* **Testosterone** and **Dihydrotestosterone**).

anesthesia   A loss of feeling or sensation. Refers to a substance given before surgery that prevents pain from being felt. *General* anesthesia causes a person to lose consciousness. Administering *local* anesthesia causes the person to remain awake, but without feeling in the area of the body where the anesthetic has been administered. *Spinal* anesthesia refers to blocking pain by injection of a local anesthetic into the space around the spinal cord.

antagonist   In medicine or medical research, an agent that nullifies the action of another agent.

antiandrogen or androgen blocker   Medication that reduces or eliminates the production or presence, and therefore the activity, of androgens.

antibiotic   A medication that is effective in killing infection-causing germs.

anus   The opening of the rectum through which solid waste leaves the body.

apex of the prostate   The tip of the prostate that is farthest away from the bladder; commonly called the *bottom of the prostate.*

asymptomatic The absence of symptoms (such as pain or fatigue) typical of a disorder such as BPH or of cancer.

atrophy A decrease in, or slow wasting away of, body tissue.

bacteria Microscopic, one-celled organisms that can, under certain conditions, cause infection.

base of the prostate Wide part of the top of the prostate, adjacent to the bladder.

benign Usually used in regard to a growth or tumor, indicating the absence of cancer; therefore, it is nonmalignant and nonrecurrent.

benign prostatic hyperplasia (BPH) The nonmalignant, abnormal multiplication of cells in the prostate gland. Commonly called *enlargement of the prostate gland,* this condition can result in the gradual compression of the urethra within the prostate, hindering urine flow. The sometimes elevated numbers in the PSA test as a result of BPH do not necessarily indicate the presence of cancer, although cancer may be present.

biopsy Removal of small samples of tissue for later microscopic examination to establish a precise diagnosis and, more specifically, to determine if cancer is present.

bladder The muscular sac, or hollow organ, that collects and stores urine in the body before it is discharged. At its fullest it can retain about a pint of urine.

bladder neck Circular muscular fibers that come together like a funnel where the bladder opens into the prostate. Constriction of the bladder neck, caused by scar tissue or prostate growth, can impede urine flow.

bone scan Viewing the bones of the body by means of a special nuclear camera. Several hours after ingestion of a substance that accumulates in abnormal bones, a picture is taken to determine if prostate cancer is present in the bones.

brachytherapy The insertion of radioactive pellets into the prostate for cancer treatment. Also called *interstitial radiation therapy.*

cancer   A cellular tumor, the natural course of which is fatal. Unlike benign tumor cells, cancer cells are capable of invading and destroying organs and of *metastasizing*—that is, of entering bodily fluids, such as blood and lymph, and thus spreading to other parts of the body.

capsule of the prostate   The fibrous tissue that comprises the outer wall of the prostate gland.

catheter   A tube inserted into a body cavity, passageway, or organ. Most commonly used for irrigation or drainage after surgery, to empty organs such as the bladder (following surgery or due to constriction), or to keep a canal open.

cell   The smallest unit of the body. All of the cells combined form all the tissues and organs of the body. When cells divide, new tissue is created.

chemotherapy   The use of specific and powerful drugs to attack and destroy cancer cells. Since they can also kill other cells in the body, chemotherapeutic agents are potentially quite dangerous.

chronic   The persistence of an illness or infection over a long period of time.

clinical trial   A planned research study to evaluate a new treatment or medication for an as yet unproven use.

complication   An unwanted, undesirable, often unpleasant, and occasionally permanent result of a treatment, procedure, or medication.

cryotherapy   Sometimes called *cryosurgery,* this term refers to using liquid nitrogen to freeze the prostate by placing probes through the perineum and into the prostate. Cryotherapy is used to eliminate cancer, but in doing so, it kills all the prostate tissue, including both cancer and normal cells.

cystoscope   An instrument composed of a slender, hollow tube with a lens at each end to allow direct visual examination of the interior of the urethra and bladder. The examination itself is called a *cystoscopy.*

deferred therapy   Another name for "watchful waiting" or delaying actual treatment but including regular monitoring.

digital rectal exam (DRE)   When a doctor inserts a gloved, lubricated finger into the rectum to feel for lumps, enlargement, or areas of hardness that might indicate the presence of cancer in the prostate. It is an exam most men dislike but one that is an important part of determining a man's health, particularly as he grows older.

dihydrotestosterone (DHT)   The more powerful hormone that results from the active breakdown of testosterone by an enzyme called 5-alpha-reductase.

diverticulum   A pouch or sac branching out from a hollow organ.

DNA (deoxyribonucleic acid)   The basic, biologically active chemical that defines the physical development and growth of humans and nearly all other living organisms.

double-blind research study   Research where neither the doctor nor the patient/subject (and sometimes the evaluator) knows which medication or treatment is being used with any individual patient. Its purpose is to minimize the effects of personal opinion or bias on the results of the study.

ejaculate   The semen expelled in a single ejaculation.

epididymis   An elongated, cordlike structure located in the testes, which stores and transmits sperm.

epithelium (or epithelial tissue)   Membranous cell tissue that covers external and internal surfaces of the body, including the lining of blood vessels and other small cavities. It is classified into several types on the basis of the number of layers of depth and the shape of the cells. Depending on where it is located, its functions include enclosing and protecting, producing secretions and excretions, and assisting in assimilation.

erectile dysfunction A more specific term for *impotence,* which refers to the inability to have and/or to maintain an erection for sexual intercourse.

external-beam radiation therapy The use of an external source, called a *linear accelerator,* to aim high-level radiation waves at a cancer.

false negative When the results of a test are erroneously reported as negative (that is, having no evidence of the condition that is being tested for) but the condition does, in fact, exist.

false positive The erroneous report of a test as positive—indicating the condition tested for does exist—when it does not, in reality, exist.

flow rate (urine) The measurement of urine as it is expelled from the bladder at its peak period of movement. A rate that is lower than normal suggests that an obstruction might be present. *See also* **peak flow rate.**

Foley catheter A catheter that is placed in the bladder for continuous drainage, usually after a prostatectomy, which may not necessarily be removed before the patient leaves the hospital. It is left in place by means of a balloon that is inflated with liquid.

Food and Drug Administration (FDA) The government regulatory agency that oversees the safety and effectiveness of new medicines and medical devices and subsequently approves, or disapproves, their distribution and use by the American public.

genitourinary tract The combination of the urinary system (kidneys, ureters, bladder, and urethra) and the genital system (including, in the male, testicles, vas deferens, prostate, and penis).

gland An aggregation or group of specialized cells that secrete or excrete materials unnecessary for their own metabolic needs but influential for the development or action of other cells and organs in the body.

hematospermia The presence of blood in the semen.

hematuria   The presence of blood in the urine.

hesitancy   When a man has to wait for several seconds or longer for his urine to flow because the bladder is straining against the resistance caused by an enlarged prostate.

hormones   Biologically active chemicals produced in the body. Hormones circulate in bodily fluids and produce a specific or stimulating effect on the activity of other cells or organs that are remote from production site cells.

hyperplasia   The abnormal enlargement of an organ or tissue because of an increase in the number of its cells.

impotence   *See* **erectile dysfunction.**

incontinence   Commonly, the leaking of urine from the bladder, but more properly called *urinary incontinence,* inasmuch as incontinence can actually mean the leaking of or inability to control any bodily substance.

inflammation   Swelling, pain, or irritation as a result of the reaction of tissue to injury or infection.

intermittency   The involuntary stopping and starting of the urinary stream due to an inability to completely empty the bladder on one single contraction.

interstitial   Situated within the spaces, or gaps in the tissue, of a particular organ.

interstitial radiation therapy   *See* **brachytherapy.**

invasive   Entry into the body by incision or by the insertion of an instrument or substance.

in vitro   Refers to studies on prostate tissue that are conducted outside a living body and in an artificial environment—usually a test tube or culture dish.

in vivo   Refers to studies on prostate tissue that remains in the living body of a human or animal while studied.

kidneys   A pair of reddish brown, bean-shaped organs embedded in fat and fibrous connective tissue and lying on either side of the spine at the base of the ribs. The left kidney tends to be slightly longer, narrower, and situated a little higher than the right kidney. Highly vascular, they are about five inches long, three inches wide, and an inch thick. The kidneys are the body's main filters. They play a pivotal role in maintaining the body's balance of fluids and electrolytes (important minerals such as sodium, potassium, and chloride); help metabolize Vitamin D; manufacture renin, which helps regulate blood pressure; and cleanse the blood of toxic wastes and excess water and salts.

luteinizing hormone-releasing hormone (LH-RH)   The hormone released by the pituitary that acts on the testes to stimulate testosterone production.

lymph   A clear fluid that drains waste from cells, traveling through vessels called *lymphatic channels* and draining into small, bean-shaped structures called *lymph nodes.*

lymph nodes   Small masses of tissue or nodules located along the vessels or channels of the lymphatic drainage system, which serves as a defense mechanism for the body by filtering and removing bacteria and other toxins (such as tumor cells). The lymph nodes are a common site for cancer spread.

malignant   Cancerous.

membrane   A thin, pliable layer of tissue that covers a surface, lines a cavity, or divides a space.

metastasis   A secondary tumor that has formed and is growing in a new site. It develops as a result of cancer cells from a first, or primary, site, traveling through the body to the second (or more) site(s).

nanograms per milliliter (ng/ml)   A minute quantity of a substance: one one-billionth of a gram (454 grams make a pound) in one one-thousandth of a liter (one liter is about a quart).

nerve-sparing prostatectomy   A refinement of prostatectomies designed in the early 1980s that saves the nerves necessary for a man to achieve penile erection. It is also called *anatomic prosta-tectomy* to distinguish it from the older style of prostatectomy, which does not save the necessary nerve bundles and which may be necessary if cancer has spread to them.

nocturia   The need to urinate frequently during the night.

oncologist   A physician specifically trained in the diagnosis and treatment of cancer.

orchiectomy   The surgical removal of one or both of the testicles. It is one way to control the development of male hormones in order to slow down the growth of prostate cancer.

palliative   Any treatment whose purpose is to relieve symptoms rather than to bring about a cure.

peak flow rate (urine)   The maximum rate of flow that a person is able to generate, measured in milliliters per second.

perineum   In a man, that part of the pelvis that is located between the bottom of the scrotum and the beginning of the anus.

placebo   Commonly used in research or clinical trials to determine the effectiveness of a drug, it is an inactive tablet that looks like the active tablet containing the medication being investigated. For the research to be a success, the active tablet must be more effective than the placebo.

postoperative or postsurgical   The time immediately after an operation and usually extending to 30 days following an operation.

primary care physician (PCP)   The first doctor to see a patient seeking medical care. This is the doctor who usually gives continuing medical care during health and illness. When an illness is beyond the expertise of the PCP, he or she will refer the patient to a specialist. In some medical plans, a patient cannot get a referral without having first consulted his or her primary care physician. Examples of primary care physicians are internists, pediatricians, family physicians, and obstetrician/gynecologists.

primary sex gland   A gland necessary for reproduction.

prostaglandin(s)   Several strong hormonelike fatty acids that act in small amounts on certain organs. In general, they are made in tiny amounts and have many different effects. They cause a variety of changes in smooth muscle tone, hormonal functions, and in the functioning of the autonomic and central nervous systems. Prostaglandins, produced by the prostate, are present in seminal fluid. They are thought to encourage the opening of the female uterus (the cervix) to dilate, making it easier for the sperm to pass into the uterus.

prostate   The walnut-shaped, muscular gland that only males have. Actually composed of muscle, connective tissue, and glandular tissue, it surrounds the urethra immediately below the bladder. The main function of the inch-and-a-half-long gland is to make part of the fluid for semen. It also provides some of the nutrient material in the semen for sperm during their journey out of the body.

prostate-specific antigen (PSA)   An enzyme secreted by the prostate gland, some of which passes into the bloodstream. Enlargement of the gland (BPH), prostatitis, and other conditions—especially cancer—can raise the level detected in the blood.

prostatic urethra   The first part of the urethra as it leaves the bladder. It is that portion of the urethra that passes through the middle of the prostate (and is therefore enclosed within it).

prostatitis   An infection of the prostate gland, usually caused by the presence of bacteria. The presence of this infection can raise the numbers of a PSA test.

prostatostasis   The most common form of nonbacterial prostatitis, generally attributed to the accumulation of excess fluid or, more specifically, to the engorgement of the prostate's fluid-producing glands due to irregular or infrequent ejaculation.

PSA   *See* **prostate-specific antigen.**

radical prostatectomy   The complete surgical removal of the prostate gland, usually done to prevent the spread of prostate cancer. *See also* **nerve-sparing prostatectomy.**

rectum   The last few inches of the intestine leading to the anus, from which waste solids leave the body.

residual urine   Any urine remaining in the bladder immediately after urination.

scrotum   The saclike structure that contains a man's testes or testicles.

secondary sex gland   A gland, such as the prostate, that is part of a person's reproductive system but is not necessary for reproduction.

semen   The thick, whitish bodily fluid that is ejaculated with orgasm. It is comprised of sperm, secretions from the prostate and other reproductive organs that carry prostaglandins (which cause strong contractions of smooth muscle), spermine (a base of several substances), fructose, glucose, citric acid, zinc, proteins, and enzymes (immunoglobulins, proteases, esterases, and phosphatase). Some elements (the sugars fructose and glucose) are thought to provide energy for the sperm, while others (zinc and many of the enzymes) may help fight disease, cleanse the urethra, and repulse attack by potentially harmful substances in the urinary tract.

seminal vesicles   Two saclike glandular structures directly behind the base of the bladder that contribute to the production of semen by secreting a fluid containing sugar and protein.

sperm or spermatozoa   The mature male germ cell that constitutes the generative element of semen and that must fertilize the female ovum for conception to take place.

staging   The process of determining the size and extent (or stage) of prostate cancer.

statistical significance   When a medical study has been conducted to determine the relative effectiveness of a certain procedure or

medication over another procedure/medication, or of no procedure at all (placebo), the conclusions generally are based on a
statistical analysis of the data (numbers) from the study. Statistical significance indicates that the results are better than those
that could have occurred by chance. It is a number—derived by
using mathematical formulas—that estimates the probability of
whether the difference in results between two groups could have
occurred by chance or is, in fact, a result of the procedure/med-
ication. There are many variables that can affect the numbers
achieved.

stricture   *See* **urethral stricture.**

stroma   In anatomy, a general term for the tissue that forms the
structural elements of an organ. It is the tissue that forms the
framework or matrix of an organ, as distinguished from the tissue that constitutes its functional element. In the prostate, stroma
is sometimes called *smooth muscle tissue* to distinguish it from
the epithelial or glandular tissue.

surgical capsule   Not really a capsule, the term is used to indicate
the point at which expanding new growth of the prostate in BPH
meets normal and true prostate tissue. During surgery for BPH,
all the tissue inside this "capsule" is removed, leaving behind
true prostatic tissue.

testes   A man's reproductive organs. Located inside the scrotum,
the testes are divided into hundreds of minuscule compartments
and are the main source of testosterone and of sperm.

testosterone   The male hormone, which comprises about 90 percent of the male hormones, or androgens, in a man's body.

transrectal ultrasound (TRUS)   The use of a probe inserted in the
rectum to produce high-frequency sound waves too high for the
human ear to hear. These sound waves are then converted into a
picture of the prostate gland and surrounding tissue.

transurethral The route through the urethra.

transurethral incision of the prostate (TUIP) A procedure involving making two incisions from the bladder neck through the prostate in order to widen the urinary passage and decrease the symptoms of BPH.

transurethral resection Removing BPH tissue that is obstructing the urethra via instruments inserted into the urethra.

transurethral resection of the prostate (TURP) A procedure for BPH wherein the surgeon tunnels through the urethra into the prostate to cut away enlarged tissue.

ultrasound *See* **transrectal ultrasound.**

ureters Fibrous, narrow, muscular tubes between 16 and 18 inches long that squeeze or milk urine from the kidneys down into the base of the bladder.

urethra A membranous canal about eight inches long that transports urine from the bladder to the exterior of the body. In men, it extends from the base of the bladder through the prostate gland (where it's called the *prostatic urethra*) into the center of the penis *(penile urethra)* and to the opening at its tip. *See also* **prostatic urethra.**

urethral stricture Scarring or narrowing within the urethra, usually caused by an injury to the urethra (as in surgery), that results in symptoms of voiding difficulty similar to those of BPH.

urinary system *See* **genitourinary tract.**

urine The fluid left over after the kidneys salvage and recycle water that passes through them. It is composed of water, sodium (salt), chloride, (the combination of chlorine and one other element), bicarbonate (soda), potassium, and urea, the breakdown product of proteins.

urodynamic studies A series of tests that yield quantitative results regarding the amounts of urine storage in the bladder and urine evacuation.

urologist   A medical doctor specially trained to deal with the medical and surgical aspects of the genitourinary tract. This is the specialist who usually diagnoses and deals with prostate cancer.

vas deferens   A tiny tube or canal about 18 inches long for carrying sperm from either testicle to the prostate gland. The two together are known as the *vasa deferentia.* When they are cut, sperm can no longer exit, so it is from them that the term *vasectomy* arises.

watchful waiting   *See* **deferred therapy.**

INDEX

A. B. Cernelle, 82, 85–86
A. B. Kabi, 82
acupuncture, low-wave frequency electrical, 22
acute bacterial prostatitis, 16–18
acute complete urinary retention, 11
Adderly, Brenda, 87, 164
aerobic exercise, 114–120
  benefits of, 117
African-American men:
  BPH, risk of, 3
  prostate cancer, risk of, 169–170
aging, and BPH development, 25
alcohol, avoiding, 155–156
alfuzosin, 61
  versus saw palmetto, 72
Allergon, 86
allium family, cancer-preventing properties of, 152–153
alpha-adrenergic blockers, 59–62, 196
alpha-blockers, 34
  disadvantage of, 77
  versus finasteride treatment, 64
alpha-tocopherol, 158
alternative medicine, suspicion of, 102–105
Alternative Therapies: Unproven Methods & Health Fraud (AMA), 103
American Association for Therapeutic Humor, 132
American Board of Medical Specialties, 111

American Medical Association (AMA):
  alternative medicine, view of, 103
  physician profiles from, 111
American Urological Association (AUA), xvi
  Symptom Score, 229–230
anal sex, and acute bacterial prostatitis, 17
Anandron, 191
Anatomy of an Illness as Perceived by the Patient: Reflections on Healing (Cousins), 131
androgen/estrogen synergism, 26
androgens, 25
  antiandrogen drugs, 190–191
  level of, 163
  and treatment procedures, 43
anecdotal reports, xiii–xiv
antagonists, 64
antihistamines, avoiding, 163
antioxidants, 119–120, 156–158
  carotenoids, 150
  in green tea, 147–148
  lycopenes, 151
  selenium, 145
anxiety, controlling, 122–129
ascorbic acid, 156–158
Asian-American men, risk of prostate cancer, 169–170

Ask-Upmark, Erik, xiii–xiv, 84
Aspund, Åke, 79–84, 87
attitude, and well-being, 136
Azuprostat, 76

balloon dilation, 51–52
Barry, M. J., 35
Beck, Aaron, 125
Becker, H., 94–95
bee pollen, 82
benign prostatic hyperplasia. *See* BPH
Berzelius, Jons Jakob, 145
beta-carotenes, 138, 150
beta-endorphins, 130
beta sitosterols, 74–76
  versus Cernitin, 93–94
Beth Israel Hospital, Center for Alternative Medicine Research, 105
Bicalutamide, 191
bioflavonoids, 148
  from ginkgo, 158
Biomarkers: The 10 Keys to Prolonging Vitality (Evans), 120
bladder:
  cancer of, 15
  infections of, 12
  neck of, contraction of, 109
  nerve damage to, 109
  obstruction of, 12
  problems with, 24
  stones, 12–13
  trabeculation of, 12–13
blood-prostate barrier, 17
blood sugar, and essential fatty acids, 142

body composition, 114
body weight, maintaining
    ideal, 120–121
Bottom Line Personal
    (newsletter), 136
Boyarsky, S., xvi
    Boyarsky scores, xvi
BPH (benign prostatic
    hyperplasia):
    absence of development,
        27–29
    annual cost of treat-
        ment, 3
    Cernitin for, 92.
        See also Cernitin
    development of, 25–27
    diagnosis of, 14–15,
        32–33
    distress from, techniques
        for decreasing, 195
    drug treatment for, 196
    lifestyle changes, influ-
        ence on, 135–164
    long-range difficulties
        of, 12–13
    versus nonbacterial
        prostatitis, 23
    Prostate Cure program
        for, 107–133
    prostate disorders,
        similarity to, 15–24
    psychological effects of,
        13–14
    risk of, and body weight,
        121
    site of, 6
    start of, 1–2
    symptom index,
        xvi–xvii
    symptoms of, 8–12
    treatment of, 33–36. *See
        also* treatment of BPH
Bräuer, H., 92–94
Burns, David, 125

cadmium, 146, 163
caffeine, avoiding,
    155–156

calories:
    burning, 113
    reducing intake of,
        144–145
Camellia sinensis, 147
cancer:
    Cernitin effect on,
        100–101
    dietary links to, 137
    in prostate, 6. *See also*
        prostate cancer
    screening for, 172
    slowest-growing type of,
        167
    unique qualities of, 179
Cardura, 61
Carlson, Richard, 129
Carlsson, Gösta, 80–84,
    86
Carter, H. Ballentine, 47
Casodex, 191
castration, and BPH devel-
    opment, 27
catastrophizing, 126–127
Center for Alternative
    Medicine Research,
    105
Centers for Disease Con-
    trol and Prevention
    (CDC), exercise rec-
    ommendations of,
    116
Cernelle, 81–82
Cernitin, 79–106, 197–198
    acceptance in United
        States, 102
    versus beta sitosterol,
        93–94
    cancer research on,
        100–101
    and complicating fac-
        tors, 99
    components of, benefi-
        cial, 87, 88
    degree of success with,
        107
    dosages of, 88–89,
        112–113

double-blind study of, 85
    drug status of, 88–89
    effectiveness of, 89–100
    FDA approval process
        for, 105–106
    versus Paraprost, 91
    Prostaphil, similarity to,
        86
    versus Tadenan, 99–100
cervix, prostaglandins and,
    5–6
chemotherapy, for prostate
    cancer, 186
cholesterol level, control-
    ling, 162
chronic bacterial prostati-
    tis, 16, 18
    depression and, 22–23
chronic pain syndrome,
    23–24
chronic prostatitis:
    Cernitin for, 92, 99
    and zinc levels, 159
cigarette smoking,
    163–165
clinical trials, xvii
    on new medications,
        66–67
cognitive therapy, 125
combined hormonal block-
    ade (CHB), 190
congestion, Cernitin effect
    on, 95
control, need for, 123
cool-down routine,
    118–119
copper intake, 161
Cousins, Norman, 131,
    135
cryotherapy, 188–189
cystitis, 12
cystoscopy, 15, 33

Debled, George, 27
decongestants, avoiding,
    163
degree of bothersomeness,
    15

depression:
  and chronic prostatitis,
    22–23
  controlling, 122–129
  DHT, 26, 28
  and enzyme inhibitors,
    62
  levels of, 170–171
diabetes, 24
diagnostic procedures,
  32–33
DIBOA, 100
diet:
  importance of, 135–136
  low-fat, 140–141,
    143–144
  for prostate health,
    121–122, 137
digital rectal exam (DRE),
  14–15, 32, 38
  annual, 172
  misdiagnosis rate of, 179
dihydrotestosterone.
  See DHT
Diokno, A. C., 52
dithiothiones, 150
diverticula, 13
Division of Cancer Pre-
  vention and Control
  of the National
  Cancer Institute, 64
doctors, selecting and
  working with,
  108–112
Dole, Bob, 182
*Don't Sweat the Small
  Stuff . . . and It's All
  Small Stuff* (Carlson),
  129
double-blind studies,
  xiv–xv
Doxazosin, 61
drugs, for treatment, 57–67
Dugan, Daniel O., 130

Ebeling, L., 94–95
ejaculation, 5–6
  retrograde, 39

electrovaporization of the
  prostate, 52–54
Ellis, Albert, 127
emotional stress, controlling, 122–129
endurance, 114
enzymatic therapy, 72
enzyme inhibitors, 62–66
epigallocatechin gallate
  (EGCG), 147–148
essential fatty acids
  (EFAs), 141–144
estrogen, and BPH devel-
  opment, 26
Eulexin, 190
Evans, William J.,
  120–121
exercise routines, 113–120
  free radicals and,
    119–120
  sample of, 119
  timing of, 113

Fair, William, 141
fat:
  body weight, percent of,
    120–121
  consumption of, and
    prostate cancer risk,
    137, 141–144, 170
fatigue, 10
fat-soluble vitamins,
  overdosing on,
  138–140
Federal Drug Administra-
  tion (FDA):
  Cernitin, approval
    process for, 105–106
  drug approval process,
    xvii
fiber, dietary, 153
finasteride, 34, 62–66
Fiore, Neil, 112, 128
fitness programs, 114
  do's and dont's of,
    114–115
5-alpha-reductase, 26
  deficiency of, 27–28

inhibitors of, 62, 67, 69,
    196
  zinc, effect on, 160
FK143, 67
flaxseed oil, 142
flexibility, 114
Flomax, 61–62
flower pollen, 80–84
flow rates, urinary, xvii
folk medicine, 103–104.
  See also alternative
    medicine
Food Guide Pyramid, 139
free radicals, 119–120,
    156–157
frequency, 13
  Cernitin effect on, 95
FR146687, 67
fruit consumption, increas-
    ing, 149–151
Fry, W. J., Jr., 131
Fujiki, H., 148
FV-7, 100–101

Galland, Leo, 108
garlic intake, 152–153
Garnick, Marc, 179
gelotology, 130
genetic deficiencies, and
    BHP development,
    27–28
genetic programming, and
    BPH development,
    26
genisten, 144
GG745, 67
ginkgo, 158–159
Gleason scoring system,
    180
glossary of terms,
    231–244
green tea, 147–149
growth factors, 26

Halpern, Steven, 124
Harzol, 75
Healing with Food
  (Webach), 159

Health Watch (newsletter), 87, 164
Healy, Bernadine, 136
Hematuria, 15
herbal supplements:
　for BPH, 67–74
　and medication, inter-
　　ference with,
　　161–162
hesitancy, 10–11
Heston, Warren, 141
high-energy transurethral
　microwave ther-
　motherapy (HE-
　TUMT), 42, 44–45
high-intensity focused
　ultrasound (HIFU),
　48
Hollander, J. B., 52
Holtgrewe, H. L., 35
hormonal therapy, for
　prostate cancer
　treatment, 189–192
hormones. *See also* testos-
　terone
　essential fatty acids for
　　production of,
　　141–142
　and fat in diet, 137,
　　140–141
　prostate cancer, links to,
　　170–171
Horney, Karen, 127
humor, physiological
　effects of, 130–133
hyperplasia, 2
Hytrin, 59–61

iatrogenic disease, 104
immune system:
　exercise, effects on, 113
　strengthening of, 136
impotence, 39
　from hormonal therapy,
　　190
　from prostate cancer
　　surgery, 181
　from prostatectomies,
　　184

from radiation treat-
　ment, 188
and TURP procedure,
　40–41
incontinence, 13, 39
　from prostate cancer
　　surgery, 181
　from prostatectomies,
　　185
intermittency, 11
International Consensus
　Committee on BPH,
　74
International Consensus on
　Urological Diseases,
　xvi–xvii
International Prostate
　Symptom Score
　(IPSS), xvii
Internet, health sites on,
　193
interstitial brachytherapy,
　188–189

Japanese men, DHT level
　of, 170–171
Jaroff, Leon, 182
*Johns Hopkins White
　Paper on Prostate
　Disorders,* 47, 154
Jönsson, Gösta, 85

Kaplan, Steven, 52
Kawamura, Nabuo, 89
Kohlmeier, Lenore, 151
Korda, Michael, 10,
　12–14, 185, 193

labeling and mislabeling,
　127
laboratory research, xiii
laser ablation, 46
laser prostatectomies, 49–51
laughter, physiological
　effects of, 130–133
Leander, Gösta, 85
LHRH therapy, 191–192
lifestyle changes affecting
　BPH, 13, 135–164

lignans, 142
linoleic and linolenic
　acids, 141–144
lipoproteins, low- and
　high-density, 162
Lupron, 190
luteinizing hormone-
　releasing hormone
　(LH-RH), 25
lycopenes, 151

Madsen-Iversen Symptom
　Severity Index, xvi
male hormones. *See* hor-
　mones; testosterone
*Man to Man: Surviving
　Prostate Cancer*
　(Korda), 185
Margolis, Simeon, 47
medical evaluation, 32
medical products, testing
　of, xiii–xvii
medication:
　for BPH treatment,
　　57–67
　and herbal preparations,
　　interference with,
　　161–162
　new, for BPH treatment,
　　66–67
mental filter, 126
Merck Research Laborato-
　ries, 28
microwave hyperthermia
　treatment:
　deep, 20
　transrectal, 21
microwave thermotherapy,
　transurethral, 21–22,
　42–45
Miller, Henry C., 18–20
minerals, 138
minipress, 61
Minter, Sue, 67
Mitscher, Lester, 147–148
moods, dealing with,
　129
muscular endurance, 114
muscular strength, 114

music, for stress relief, 124

Nagakubo, Ichiron, 89
National Institute of Diabetes and Digestive and Kidney Disease (NIDDK), 26–27
National Institute of Health, Office of Alternative Medicine, 105
needle biopsies, 178
negativity, 124–128
neurological disorders, 24
nilutamide, 191
nocturia, Cernitin effect on, 95, 96
nonbacterial prostatitis, 16, 19, 23
    versus stress prostatitis, 18–21

Office of Alternative Medicine, 105
Ohkoshi, Masaaki, 89
Omega-3 (linolenic acid), 141–144
Omega-6 (linoleic acid), 141–144
Ornish, Dean, 136
outflow obstruction, Cernitin for, 98
overgeneralization, 126

Palmstierna, Hans, 83
Paraprost, 91–92
perineum, 20
Permixon, 69
personalization, 128
pharmacotherapy, 57–67
phytochemicals, 150
phytoesterols, 74–75
phytopharmaceutical agents, 68–74
phytosterols, 73
pilot studies, xiv
placebos, xiv

plant extracts, for BPH treatment, 67–74
polarized thinking, 125–126
Pollendragées, 82–83
Pollisan, 80–82
Pollitabs, 83
polyphenols, EGCG, 148
positive experiences, disqualifying, 126
prazosin, 61
    versus saw palmetto, 72
primary care physicians, 109–110
Pritikin, Nathan, 136
prolactin, 160
Proscar, 28, 62–66
    effectiveness of, measuring, 76–77
    versus *Serenoa repens,* 70–71
prostaglandins, 5–6
    inhibitors of, 152–153
Prostaphil, 86
prostate:
    digital rectal exam of, 14–15. *See also* digital rectal exam
    disorders of, 3, 15–24
    enlargement of, 3, 6–7, 38
    lobes of, 6
    role of, 4–8
    zinc, use of, 159–160
prostate cancer, 11–12, 24–25, 165–193
    action against, 192–193
    body weight and, 121
    causes of, probable, 168–171
    and Cernitin, 100–101
    and cigarette smoking, 163–164
    dietary links to, 137
    evaluation and diagnosis, 178–179
    exercise, effect on, 119–120

grading of, 180–181
    and green tea intake, 149
    hormonal therapy for, 189–192
    and low-fat diets, 140
    metastatic sites for, 179–180
    obesity and, 121
    PSA test screening for, 171–173
    screening for, and finasteride treatment, 63–64
    and selenium intake, 145
    statistics of, 166
    treatment of, 181–192
    and Vitamin D production, 154
    watchful waiting for, 182–183
Prostate Cancer Prevention Trial (PCPT), 64–66
prostatectomies, 35, 38–39. *See also* surgery
    laser, 49–51
    perineal, 51
    radical, 183–186
    transurethral resection of prostate, 39–41
Prostate Cure program, 107–133
prostate-specific antigen (PSA), 63–64, 93
    free, 175–177
    rate of change in, 177
    rise in, 173–174
    test, 167–168, 171–177, 179
prostatic acid phosphatase (PAP), 93
    test, 180–181
prostatic fluid, 5–6
prostatism, 11–12
prostatitis, 16
    and Cernitin, 84
    stress, 19–24

prostatodynia, 16, 19
    Cernitin for, 99
    versus stress prostatitis,
        20–21
prostatostasis, 18
protein intake, effects of,
    149–150
psychological difficulties:
    and chronic prostatitis,
        22–23
    and nonbacterial prosta-
        titis, 23
pumpkin seeds, 68
Pygeum africanum extract,
    72–74

quality of life, and TUMT
    treatment, 43
Quality of Life scale, xvii

radiation therapy, for
    prostate cancer,
    186–189
radical prostatectomy,
    183–186
randomization, xv
*Reader's Guide to Alterna-
    tive Health Methods*
    (AMA), 103
Recommended Daily
    Allowance (RDA),
    139
rectal coil magnetic
    resonance imaging
    (MRI), 32
Reference Daily Intake
    (RDI), 139
relaxation, making time
    for, 122–124
residual urine volume,
    Cernitin effect on, 95
Rippe, James, 113, 115
Rosenfeld, Isadore,
    143–144
Rous, Stephen N., 4, 188
rye pollen, 68

Sabal serrulata, 69
Salcedo, Hernando, 20

Salmon, J. Warren, 104
saw palmetto berry extract,
    68–72
    versus alfuzosin, 72
    versus prazosin, 72
Schachter, Michael, 27
Schwarzkopf, H. Norman,
    173–174, 178
Scientific Committee of
    the First International
    Consultation on BPH,
    71
scientific studies, xiv
selenium, 145–146
seminal fluid, 5–6
Serenoa repens extract,
    68–72
    versus Proscar, 70–71
serum creatinine level, 32
sexual activity, and BPH,
    3–4
sexual difficulties, and
    BPH, 14. *See also*
    impotence
Shapiro, Charles E., 73–74
"should" statements, 127
side effects, of BPH
    symptoms, 10
single-blind studies, xv
smoking, avoiding or
    quitting, 163–164
soy-based foods, 144
sperm, prostatic fluid and,
    5–6
spicy foods, avoiding,
    155–156
Stanford University,
    Center for Research
    in Disease Preven-
    tion, 105
stasis, 12
stents, 54
stinging nettle root, 68,
    74
stress:
    controlling, 122–129
    and prostatitis, 19–20
stress prostatitis, 19–24
stretching, 118–119

subjective experience, of
    patients, 104, 192.
    See also alternative
    medicine
subjective reasoning, 127
sulforaphane, 151
Suramin, 191
surgeons, selecting,
    111–112
surgery, 37–39. *See also*
    prostatectomies
    open, 51
    transurethral incision of
        prostate, 41–42
    transurethral micro-
        wave thermotherapy,
        42–45
    transurethral resectomy
        of prostate, 39–41
surgical capsule, 38
symptoms:
    categorizing, xvi
    indexes of, xvi–xvii
Symptom Score, 230

Tadenan, 73
    versus Cernitin, 99–100
Talso, 69
Tammela, Teuvo, 41
Tamsulosin, 61–62
Te, Alexis, 52
Terazosin, 59
testosterone, 25–26
    blocking, 190–191
    and BPH development,
        25
    decreased levels of,
        26–27
    and diet, 137
thermotherapy, 46
    transurethral microwave,
        42–45
Tobishi Pharmaceutical
    Co., Ltd., Cernitin
    study by, 89–90
tomatoes, beneficial
    effects of, 151–152
Tonisson, E. P., 83
trabeculation, 12–13

transitional zone, as site of
    BPH, 6
transrectal ultrasound
    (TRUS), 32, 178–179
transurethral balloon laser
    thermotherapy
    (TUBAL-T), 50–51
transurethral dilation,
    51–52
transurethral incision of
    the prostate (TUIP),
    41–42
transurethral laser vapor-
    ization (TUVP),
    49–50
transurethral microwave
    thermotherapy
    (TUMT), 42–45
transurethral needle abla-
    tion (TUNA), 45–47
transurethral resection of
    the prostate (TURP),
    38–41, 196–197
    annual number per-
        formed, 58
    versus transurethral
        microwave thermo-
        therapy, 43–44
transurethral ultrasound-
    guided laser-induced
    prostatectomy
    (TULIP), 49
treatment of BPH, 33–36
    annual costs of, 3
    with beta-sitosterols,
        74–76
    developing techniques,
        52–54
    direct costs of, 35
    with drugs, 57–67
    effectiveness measures,
        xvii
    with herbal supple-
        ments, 67–74
    HIFU, 48

laser prostatectomies,
    49–51
outdated methods, 51–52
surgery, 37–39
TUIP, 41–42
TUMT, 42–45
TUNA, 45–47
TURP, 39–41
watchful waiting, 36–37
Tyler, Varro, 162

urethra, 5
    and prostate, 8
    scarring or stricture of,
        24, 109
urinalysis, 32
urinary flow rate, xvii
urinary frequency, 13, 95
urinary tract:
    diet for health of,
        121–122
    obstruction of, 8–12
    prostate and, 7–8
urination:
    difficulty in, 10–11
    discomfort, at end of, 20
    dribbling, at end of, 11
    false need to, 10
urine:
    blood in, 15
    residual, 33, 95
    retention of, and water
        intake volume,
        146–147
urologists, 109–110
Urtica dioica root, 68, 74

Vane, J. R., 142
vas deferens, 6
vasectomies, and risk of
    prostate cancer, 171
vegetable consumption,
    increasing, 149–151
vegetarianism, and hor-
    mone levels, 170

visual laser ablation of the
    prostate (VLAP),
    49–50
Vitamin A deficiencies, 151
Vitamin C, 156–158
Vitamin D, 154–155
Vitamin E, 138, 158
vitamin supplements,
    138–140

walking, for exercise,
    115–118
Walsh, Patrick C., 173,
    181
    radical prostatectomy,
        refining of, 184
warm-up routines,
    118–119
watchful waiting, 34, 36–37
    for prostate cancer treat-
        ment, 182–183
water intake, 146–147
website pages, for clinical
    trial information and
    innovations, 52
weight-bearing exercise,
    118–119
Werbach, Melvyn,
    159–160
Whitaker, Julian, 71
white American men:
    BPH, risk of, 3
    prostate cancer, risk of,
        169
"why me" questions,
    dwelling on, 128
workouts. See exercise
    routines

Xafral, 61

Young, H. H., 172

zinc, 159–161
Zoladex, 190–191

Dear Reader:

Thank you for buying my latest book, *The Prostate Cure*. My specialty is researching and writing about health topics, and I'm just as cynical as you about information based on rumor and hype. That's why, in my newsletter, just as in this book, I'll bring you honest, fully supported research to help you separate the facts from the fiction. In upcoming issues, I'll provide convincing information on the following topics:

- Innovative ways to boost your energy—naturally
- Enhancing your sex drive and saying no to Viagra
- Updates on pain relief for arthritis sufferers
- Exciting new weight-loss supplements
- Invigorating an aging or failing memory

Because I know you care about your health, I'm offering you the chance to receive a *no-risk* trial subscription to my monthly newsletter, *Health Watch*. Order today, and start living a better, healthier life. If at any time you are not completely satisfied with my newsletter, you may simply cancel your subscription and receive a full refund.

As a preferred reader and someone who has already purchased one of my books, I'm offering this *no-risk* one-year trial subscription for only $36.95— or 38% off the regular subscription price of $59.95.

Healthfully yours,

Brenda D. Adderly

To order your NO-RISK trial subscription to my monthly *Health Watch* newsletter, call 1-888-211-2800, or send in the form below!

❏ YES! Please sign me up for my NO-RISK trial subscription to Health Watch for only $36.95 for 12 issues. I understand that I may cancel my subscription at any time and receive a full refund. Mail this card to: Alter-Net Health Technologies, 144 N. Robertson Blvd, Suite 103, Los Angeles, CA 90048. Allow 4 weeks for delivery.

❏ Visa   ❏ MC   ❏ AmEx   Expiration date: _____

Account no. _____

Please print: Mr./Mrs./Ms. _____

Address _____

City _____   State _____   Zip _____

Your signature _____